Clinical Assessment of Human Suffering

Ana Claudia de Lima Quintana Arantes

Clinical Assessment of Human Suffering

Planning Care in the End of Life

Springer

Ana Claudia de Lima Quintana Arantes
Association Casa do Cuidar
São Paulo
Brazil

ISBN 978-3-030-57533-5   ISBN 978-3-030-57535-9 (eBook)
https://doi.org/10.1007/978-3-030-57535-9

This Springer imprint is published by the registered company Springer Nature Switzerland AG
The registered company address is: Gewerbestrasse 11, 6330 Cham, Switzerland

Preface

The purpose of this book is to assist doctors and other health care professionals involved in assessment, care planning, and patient assistance at the end-of-life stage. It provides a unique and humanistic view of the challenges of good palliative care practice. Concepts and definitions, resources and therapeutic alternatives, patients' symptoms, and the assessment of physical, emotional, family, social, and spiritual dimensions are addressed in a clear and practical way, demystifying and dissolving the barriers and difficulties encountered in palliative care. The dimensions of the human being are many and complementary. Often, a cure for a physical ailment does not entail the absence of suffering. Undergoing aggressive treatments is also a source of great suffering. Thus, the approach of the work of multidimensional care for human suffering can promote a clearer understanding for the patient, their family, and mainly the physician and the assistance team who will promote this care.

Contents

Chapter 1
Introduction

I really like this picture. It depicts the moment of waiting for a meeting. Of the doctor with the patient. Of the caregiver with the person who needs care. Pay attention to the picture: note that the patient has made preparations for this visit. As she is being treated in a country in serious trouble with its population's health, she must have waited a few months for this meeting. Possibly, this appointment will not last much longer than a few minutes—maybe 10, maybe 15 minutes. She waits, watchful and ready: she has chosen a gorgeous outfit, earrings, and hat. She has her glasses carefully in place, looking at the empty chair in front of her. What goes on in her mind probably concerns everything she needs to ask, knowing she will have the shortest amount of time to have her doubts resolved. She has an intense trajectory of suffering—AIDS and lymphoma. She does not know it yet, but when the doctor comes in, they will have the painful mission of informing her that the disease is back, unmerciful and with no chances of treatment. All possibilities of intervention have been exhausted and failed. My question is: has the person who is going to sit in front of this woman prepared to appreciate these 15 minutes that will change her life in a direction no one is ready to follow: suffering—and death? (Fig. 1.1)

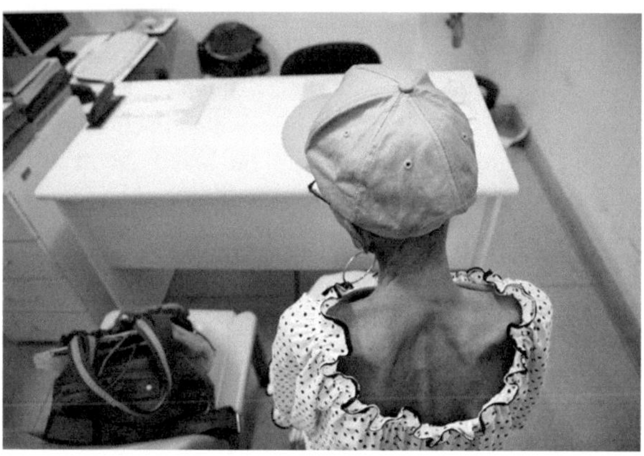

Fig. 1.1 The moment of waiting for a meeting of the patient with the doctor

A. C. L. Q. Arantes, *Clinical Assessment of Human Suffering*,
https://doi.org/10.1007/978-3-030-57535-9_1

For this reason, we have come to this book and its content: it is necessary to prepare health care professionals for this meeting so they know how to evaluate the suffering of someone who is close to reaching the end of their life, so they know how to approach and diagnose this suffering in all of its dimensions and complexities. Through a watchful and detailed evaluation, the decisions concerning how to approach and treat each of the dimensions—biological, emotional, family, social, and spiritual—will have much better chances of achieving the best result possible.

There comes a time in which we worry about having a checkup, losing the muffin top, taking care of life, taking care of the kids. Thinking about death makes us think something has to be done. Another serious mistake is that we distance ourselves from "being" by way of "doing"; then we think a good life is a life that has led us to have things and do things. But when the time comes for illness, there is nothing we can do anymore. And when we stop doing, we think this is dying—but not quite yet. The idea of "being" human is simply existing and making a difference where we are, for being who we are. People who are absent from their own lives will just be "absences" in their time of dying. Many people are like that in life, an almost constant absence. And when they are present, we feel that this time is empty.

Coming back to the dimensions of death, in order to help a dying person, it is necessary to understand what is happening with them. The biological dimension is a necessary condition only for the other dimensions to express themselves. We are all complex beings, men or women, children or elderly, of any color, race, creed, or beliefs. We are beings who contemplate the possibility of valuing our physical dimension because we are here, in this time and place. We also have an emotional dimension, the most universal there is—universal in the sense of size, of complexity, not in the conception that it is the same for everyone. Then there are the family dimension and the social dimension.

I can nearly say that almost all articles and studies concerning the dimensions of suffering reckon there are four: physical, emotional, social, and spiritual. As I have been working in this area for a long time, I have allowed myself to separate the social dimension from the family dimension. Family dynamics have complexities that do not depend on the society in which one lives. Each family is its own microcosm, whose functioning may be either good or bad. An approach to family suffering allowing free expression of the perceptions, expectations, beliefs, and values of all involved leads to consolidation of a stronger support network for the patient. We need to understand that the suffering of each member will be lived and expressed within the biography shared with the loved one in suffering, and that this expression is also going to depend on the possibility of experiencing anticipatory grief (this is better explained in the chapter on grief).

The whole process of evaluation of suffering in all of its dimensions takes the health care professional to a space of higher understanding of care priorities and better planning of modular actions with the goal of symptom relief and management.

Globally, more than 56.8 million people are estimated to require palliative care every year. The majority (67.1%) are adults over 50 years old and at least 7% are children. The majority (54.2%) are non-decedents who need palliative care prior to their last year of life. The burden of severe illness and health related suffering, and the corresponding need for palliative care, are immense [1, 2]. Palliative care improves the quality of life of patients and their families who face problems associated with life-threatening illnesses—whether physical, psychosocial, or spiritual—yet palliative care is still not accessible by most people in need, especially in low and middle-income countries (LMICs). The majority of adults in need of palliative care (76%) live in LMICs, and the highest proportion are in countries of low-income. Non-communicable diseases account for almost 69% of adult need. Among adults, the illnesses and conditions that generate most serious suffering requiring palliative care interventions are cancer, HIV/AIDS, cerebrovascular, dementias, and lung diseases. Overly restrictive regulations for prescribing and accessing morphine and other essential controlled drugs deny these people access to adequate pain relief and quality palliative care. The ability to offer adequate pain relief throughout the course of a life-threatening illness is one of the purposes of palliative care described by the World Health Organization [3].

The global need for palliative care will continue to grow as a result of the growing burden of noncommunicable diseases and an aging population. Early palliative care reduces unnecessary hospitalizations and the use of health services. As defined by the World Health Organization in 2017 [4]:

> Palliative care is an approach that improves the quality of life of patients and their families facing the problem associated with life-threatening illness, through the prevention and relief of suffering by means of early identification and impeccable assessment and treatment of pain and other problems, physical, psychosocial and spiritual.

Dr. Eric Cassell [5], in a text on the diagnosis of suffering, tells us:

> The alleviation of suffering is crucial in all of medicine, especially in the care of the dying. Suffering cannot be treated unless it is recognized and diagnosed. Suffering involves some symptom or process that threatens the patient because of fear, the meaning of the symptom, and concerns about the future. The meanings and the fear are personal and individual, so that even if two patients have the same symptoms, their suffering would be different. The complex techniques and methods that physicians usually use to make a diagnosis, however, are aimed at the body rather than the person.

The information on which the assessment of suffering is based generally follows a subjective perspective, and this may pose a great challenge, especially for physicians. The relief of human suffering depends on physicians who acquire skills in assessing human suffering in a multidimensional fashion.

References

1. Connor SR, editor. Global Atlas of Palliative Care. London; 2020. http://www.thewhpca.org/resources/global-atlas-on-end-of-life-care. Accessed 20 Nov 2020.
2. World Health Organization. Palliative care. Geneva: World Health Organization; 2018. https://www.who.int/news-room/fact-sheets/detail/palliative-care. Accessed 10 Aug 2020.
3. Wright M, Wood J, Lynch T, Clark D. Mapping levels of palliative care development: a global view. Lancaster: Lancaster University; 2006. Accessed 10 Aug 2020.
4. World Health Organization. WHO definition of palliative care. Geneva: World Health Organization; 2017. https://www.who.int/cancer/palliative/definition/en/. Accessed 10 Aug 2020.
5. Cassell EJ. Diagnosing suffering: a perspective. Ann Intern Med. 1999;131(7):531–4. https://doi.org/10.7326/0003-4819-131-7-199910050-00009. Accessed 10 Aug 2020.

Chapter 2
The Multidimensional Human Being

Humans beings are complex beings, gifted with multiple impressions regarding the world and themselves, learned and incorporated into their way of living and thinking throughout their lives. At birth, we are essentially a biological being, but as we grow older, our biographical dimension is enriched. And our suffering dimension goes way beyond suffering from physical illness. Cats are born cats, and each one believes it is the only one to exist, for it does not know the stories of other cats. If it gets sick, it has no sense of suffering from finitude, because it is oblivious to the natural history of life.

As human beings grow, we learn stories of the lives of other human beings. Some diseases already have a well-recorded history in the collective unconscious as facades of the end of life. Just knowing about a diagnosis—of cancer, for example—makes us think about the threat to our integrity. Other diseases still in disguise, such as diabetes and heart failure, carry in themselves great gravity but cover up their importance and deprive their carriers of knowing how much they can threaten them (Fig. 2.1).

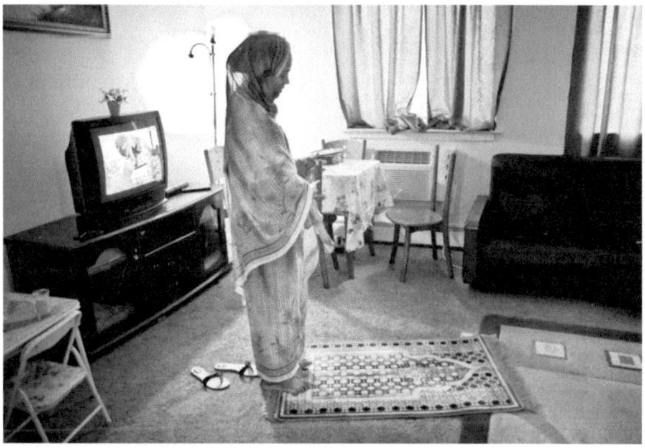

Fig. 2.1 Throughout their lives, human beings learn and incorporate emotional, family, social, professional, existential, and spiritual dimensions

A. C. L. Q. Arantes, *Clinical Assessment of Human Suffering*,
https://doi.org/10.1007/978-3-030-57535-9_2

The dimensions of the human being are many and complementary. Emotional, family, social, professional, existential, and spiritual dimensions are, in fact, the true marks that define who we really are. Our differences are not defined only by our DNA. Therefore, in case there is no chance of dissociating a diseased organ from the organism that houses it, we have to accept that we must take care of the human being as a whole, so the cure can also be achieved as a whole. When we suffer from any physical ailment, all of our being responds to this suffering. Emotionally, socially, and spiritually, we reflect our physical ill-being.

And, often, the cure of a physical ailment does not imply the absence of suffering.

A disease can impose varying degrees of suffering, depending on how much it interferes with life as a whole. The exact moment we are given the diagnosis of a disease that threatens the continuity of our life is, in itself, an instant of great suffering. We then undergo many moments of re-evaluation of our priorities and the fundamental truths that must really guide us in life. Undergoing aggressive treatments that can take away the quality time we still have left is also a source of great suffering.

Palliative care offered to people diagnosed with serious illness that threatens the continuity of life can have a significant impact on quality of life, to the point of influencing the life expectancy. The focus of palliative care is the treatment of suffering, seeking to fulfill the needs of the human being as a whole, with relief of physical symptoms occasioned by the illness or its treatment. Emotional, social, and spiritual comfort are also part of the active context of palliative care and have proved themselves ever more fundamental in the alleviation of suffering. We can identify—through the clinical history and careful physical examination, and even utilizing laboratory and imaging resources—the functioning and anatomy of organs and biological systems. But we are not capable of measuring the level of fear or guilt that runs in the blood along with tumor markers or sugar levels. We are not able to tell how much infiltration of sorrow and rejection may be present in the functioning of each organ that suffers from serious illness. That is why making use of resources provided by social services and psychology teams—trained to identify suffering that is intangible, immense, and not measurable in a laboratory—makes a world of difference in the quality of care.

In the palliative care approach, the greatest will is the patient's, and their voice is the one that governs and determines the direction of care. Therefore, a well-conducted assessment is the first and most fundamental step toward the success of this work. An insufficient or imprecise evaluation can result in a succession of errors and mistakes in diagnostic or therapeutic procedures. And since a person's time is precious, especially at the end of life, an error in approach bleeds important moments that can never return. We are multidimensional beings. We will never be just a body or a disease. We have our history and our biography, and in this biography we have our faces, composed of broad dimensions that characterize us:

1. The body, in its biological dimension—which makes us feel the internal world. When bearing a serious disease, the body starts to express signs and symptoms of discomfort, which make it difficult or impossible for us to achieve a sense of well-being.

2. The feelings, in their emotional dimension—which make us experience what our internal and external worlds offer us. Faced with a threat to the integrality of being, this dimension can be a way of reorganizing us in the face of this possibility of death, but it can also be the main agent of our greatest suffering.
3. Intimate relationships, in their family dimension—which characterize us as gregarious beings, making us feel part of an important group.
4. Supporting relationships, in their social dimension.
5. The essence of the human being, in its spiritual dimension.

We believe it is the physician's duty to understand that suffering is more feared than death and that it is a priority to provide comfort and relief from pain and other symptoms that cause identifiable suffering.

2.1 Principles of Palliative Care

According to the World Health Organization (WHO) [1–3], the principles of palliative care are as follows:

1. *Provide impeccable control of pain and stressful symptoms.* The effort dedicated to reducing the measurements of a tumor, using all available techniques and protocols in order to obtain this result, should be applied at the same intensity when we encounter a patient who complains of pain. The complaint of fatigue—considered by patients, doctors, and family members as one of the most stressful symptoms of the disease and oncological treatment—is hardly treated properly. The vast majority of doctors are limited to instructing the patient to rest. With this guidance, the physician instigates progressive worsening of symptoms, leading to physical deconditioning that is difficult to reverse. The same problem applies to the complaint of insomnia [4]: although we have evidence that significant sleep deprivation can significantly impair the benefits of cancer treatment, the prescription of corticosteroids at inappropriate times persists in chemotherapy and other pharmaceutical prescriptions.
2. *Do not use resources that shorten the life-span, and do not use futile therapies that lead to prolongation of human suffering.* The relationship established between the use of opioids and a reduced life-span is very common in society in general. However, we already have studies in the literature that demonstrate greater survival in patients who receive palliative care. Some studies have shown a survival increase of up to 29 days, with the least possible suffering, in patients cared for in hospices [5]. For patients with an early diagnosis, the decrease in the quality of life caused by uncontrolled symptoms can lead to a significant impairment of life expectancy [6].
3. *Offer a support system that allows the patient to live as actively as possible.* Palliative care provides the patient and their family with the certainty of a com-

mitment to quality of life and achievement of goals that are consistent with the reality of each patient. Individualized treatment can favor an active, quality life, even in situations of irreversible disease.
4. *Offer a family support system that allows an accurate understanding of the disease process in all phases.* The family is also an important focus of palliative care activities. We all have families. Nuclear families may be small or even non-existent, but "expanded" families, which include more distant relatives and friends, are part of our life, and their suffering must also be considered when we are facing a clear situation of finitude. The support and guidance provided by palliative care can be decisive in maintaining serenity in the final moments of a human being.
5. *Integrate psychological and spiritual aspects into the work of caring.* Attribution of importance to the patient's emotional and spiritual aspects favors elaboration of the reality of finitude, as it constitutes the core of a meaning that can be construed only from this recognition. Spirituality is an essential characteristic of the human being, because only this species can give meaning to its existence. An elephant cannot question itself about the "why" of being an elephant, but a man can spend a lifetime with this question in his mind. When we find a sense that "transcends" our reality, we face our "spirituality." Several studies have shown that spirituality is valued by patients and family members, and can be an independent factor in quality of life [7, 8].
6. *Joint efforts by a multidisciplinary team offer the most comprehensive care possible.*
7. *An improvement in quality of life can positively influence the patient's lifespan* [4, 5].

2.2 The Care Plan

2.2.1 The Biological Dimension

- Pain control
- Weakness and fatigue management
- Sleep
- Gastrointestinal complaints
- Skin care and oral hygiene
- Care for secretions and odors
- Diagnosis and management of delirium
- Incontinence
- Dyspnea and other respiratory symptoms
- Dry membranes

2.2.2 *The Emotional Dimension*

- Sadness
- Rage
- Fear
- Blame
- Feelings of helplessness or abandonment
- Loss of control
- Major depression
- Anxiety

2.2.3 *The Social/Family Dimension*

- Citizens rights: tax relief and payouts from unemployment insurance, guarantee funds, etc. Guidance from a social worker is required.
- Caring for families: detecting risk of family fatigue or exhaustion of the main caregiver.
- Detailed guidance on symptom management and patient care when the patient wants to stay at home.
- Support in elaboration of the care and needs of the family and home caregivers.
- Support in the division of tasks previously performed by the patient.

2.2.4 *The Spiritual Dimension*

The spiritual approach must necessarily involve unconditional respect for the beliefs and values of each patient and their family [7, 8]. The presence of a spiritual adviser (chaplain) would be ideally conceived, but, in the absence of one, the recommendation of the health team regarding the appropriateness of involving a spiritual adviser or a religious leader can favor the resolution of several types of suffering related to this human dimension.

2.3 Diversity of Individual Experiences of Suffering

The perception of discomfort and disease burden among patients in palliative care is highly individual. To address the complexity of suffering, Dame Cicely Saunders, the founder of modern hospices and palliative care, coined the term "total pain." Saunders noted that her patients' pain included not only the physical aspect but also emotional and mental suffering, social problems, and a spiritual need for security and meaning [9]. Consequently, the concept of total pain, which provides a defining structure for the assessment of patients in palliative care, refers to the complex mechanisms and manifestations of suffering, including its physical, emotional, socioeconomic, and spiritual components.

A person's pain or malaise, their body image, their feelings about their illness, their desires, their relationships, and their spiritual values or beliefs contribute to their experience of illness and suffering [10]. However, no accurate clinical taxonomy of suffering is available [11], because total pain is constructed in a highly individual manner. There is no single, good way to deal with a serious illness; likewise, there is no single definition of what constitutes a "good" death [12].

Given the diversity of the individual experience of suffering, the specific needs and objectives of palliative care for individual patients are challenging to identify a priori or derive from population studies [13].

References

1. World Health Organization. Cancer pain relief and palliative care. Geneva: WHO; 2004.
2. World Health Organization. Symptom relief in terminal illness. Geneva: World Health Organization; 1998. https://apps.who.int/iris/handle/10665/42121. Accessed 10 Aug 2020.
3. Davies E, Higginson IJ. The solid facts: palliative care. Copenhagen: WHO Regional Office for Europe; 2004. https://apps.who.int/iris/handle/10665/107561. Accessed 10 Aug 2020.
4. Connor S, Pyenson B, Fitch K, Spence C, Iwasaki K. Comparing hospice and non-hospice patient survival among patients who die within a three-year window. J Pain Symptom Manag. 2007;33(3):238–46. https://doi.org/10.1016/j.jpainsymman.2006.10.010.
5. Lis CG, Gupta D, Granick J, Grutsch JF. Can patient satisfaction with quality of life predict survival in advanced colorectal cancer? Support Care Cancer. 2006;14(11):1104–10. https://doi.org/10.1007/s00520-006-0100-3.
6. Puchalski CM, Dorff RE, Hendi IY. Spirituality, religion, and healing in palliative care. Clin Geriatr Med. 2004;20(4):689–714, vi–vii. https://doi.org/10.1016/j.cger.2004.07.004.
7. Puchalski C. Caregiver stress: the role of spirituality in the lives of family/friends and professional caregivers. In: Carter R, editor. Caregiving book series. Americus: Rosalynn Carter Institute for Human Development, Georgia Southwestern State University; 2003.
8. Doyle D, Hanks GW, Macdonald N. Oxford textbook of palliative medicine. 2nd ed. Oxford: Oxford University Press; 1998.
9. Saunders C. The depths and the possible heights. Medical News; 1964. p. 16–17.
10. Wilson KG, Chochinov HM, McPherson CJ, LeMay K, Allard P, Chary S, Gagnon PR, Macmillan K, De Luca M, O'Shea F, Kuhl D, Fainsinger RL. Suffering with advanced cancer. J Clin Oncol. 2007;25(13):1691–7. https://doi.org/10.1200/JCO.2006.08.6801.
11. Cassell EJ. Recognizing suffering. Hastings Cent Rep. 1991;21(3):24–31.
12. Steinhauser KE, Christakis NA, Clipp EC, McNeilly M, McIntyre L, Tulsky JA. Factors considered important at the end of life by patients, family, physicians, and other care providers. JAMA. 2000;284(19):2476–82. https://doi.org/10.1001/jama.284.19.2476.
13. Munday D, Petrova M, Dale J. Exploring preferences for place of death with terminally ill patients: qualitative study of experiences of general practitioners and community nurses in England. BMJ. 2009;339:b2391. https://doi.org/10.1136/bmj.b2391.

Chapter 3
Oncological Disease Versus Nononcological Disease: Differences and Similarities in Their Manifestations of Suffering

3.1 Prognostic Evaluation

In the roots of medical practice there was a certain harmony between science and the mystical priesthood, which surrounded the physician's powers to evaluate and cure illness. Nevertheless, the art of predicting the future has not yet become sufficiently scientific to the point of specializing the physician in the exercise of prognosis. This evaluation seeks constant support from use of scales, signs, and symptoms that may identify the death process at the early stages, but it still involves rather complex physiological and social resolutions. Even though death is a clearly identified biological phenomenon, the perceptions of meaning, time, and circumstances in which the process of dying is succeeded by death still remain weakly established and weakly taught knowledge. The greatest danger of this exercise of evaluating a person's survival is determining "social" death before physical death itself. Once it has been established that a patient has a short life expectancy, estimated in days or weeks, we are at risk of underestimating their needs and neglecting the possibility of real comfort within the patient's and their family's evaluation. In general, the prognostic evaluation of patients at advanced stages of serious illness still presents considerable optimistic error, especially during evaluation of patients with nonneoplastic disease. A 2000 study by Christakis and Lamont [1] demonstrated that the accuracy of prognoses generally erred on the side of optimism. Only 20% of physicians made accurate predictions (within 33% of their patients' actual survival time), whereas 63% were overoptimistic and 17% underestimated survival. An interesting conclusion was that the longer the duration of the doctor–patient relationship was, the lower the prognosis accuracy was, demonstrating that the bond established between a physician and their patient determined a "wish" by the physician to predict the patient's condition, implying a diminished capacity to evaluate the reality (Fig. 3.1). This finding allows us to initiate a pertinent discussion about whether the physician's own wishes and expectations might interfere in their evaluation of their patient's prognosis. One of the tools available to us in prognostic evaluation

A. C. L. Q. Arantes, *Clinical Assessment of Human Suffering*,
https://doi.org/10.1007/978-3-030-57535-9_3

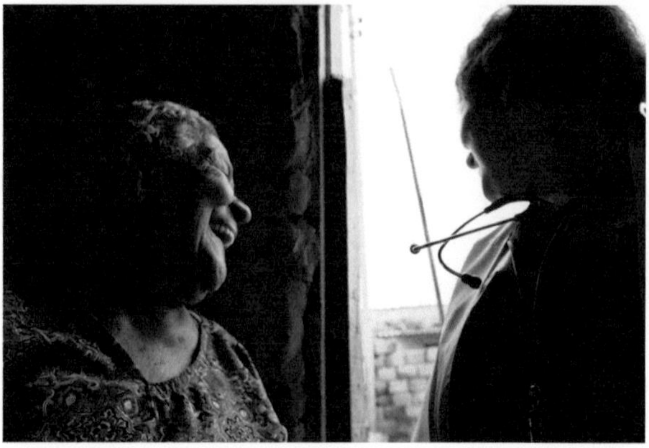

Fig. 3.1 The bond established between a physician and their patient may affect the accuracy of the prognosis estimated by the physician

Table 3.1 Main functional dependencies

Basic activities of daily living
Urinary and fecal incontinence
Feeding through enteral tubes or inability to feed/hydrate without assistance
Permanent immobilization in a bed or on an armchair

measures the patient's functional capacity. However, we know that functional capacity may be directly related to a condition of intense suffering that is evaluated or treated inadequately, and that distorts prognostic evaluation. For instance, a patient with prostate cancer could be compromised in his functionality because of severe bone pain that is left untreated, and not by systemic deterioration caused by his underlying condition. In this case, the systemic deterioration would be due to suffering and not the progression of the disease to vital organs. As for evaluating the capacity for daily activities, we have palliative care recommendations for patients who depend on others for certain activities because of inability to move, inability to feed, or incontinence (Table 3.1).

3.2 How to Measure Functional and Clinical Decline

The Karnofsky Performance Status Scale (Table 3.2) has been developed for cancer patients as an objective means of documenting the patient's clinical decline and evaluating their capacity to accomplish certain basic activities. Most patients with a Karnofsky score lower than 70% qualify for palliative care, unless ongoing treatment for the underlying condition is available, bearable, and expected to be beneficial. Another useful instrument for measuring the patient's clinical condition is the Palliative Performance Scale (Table 3.3), which was developed in 1996 in Victoria (British Columbia, Canada) and revised in 2001.

Table 3.2 Karnofsky Performance Status Scale

Level (%)	Comments
100	Normal, no complaints, no evidence of disease
90	Able to carry on normal activity, minor signs or symptoms of disease
80	Normal activity with effort, some signs or symptoms of disease
70	Cares for self, unable to carry on normal activity or to do active work
60	Requires occasional assistance but is able to care for most of [their] needs
50	Requires considerable assistance and frequent medical care
40	Disabled, requires special care and assistance
30	Severely disabled, hospitalization is indicated although death not imminent
20	Hospitalization necessary, very sick, active supportive treatment necessary
10	Moribund, fatal processes progressing rapidly
0	Dead

Reproduced from Karnofsky and Burchenal

To circumvent the difficulty of prognostic evaluation, some clinical criteria have been established for each illness or each clinical condition, which support the decision on referral to palliative care. Some of these criteria relate to specific morbid conditions, such as congestive heart failure, chronic obstructive pulmonary disease (COPD), cancer, amyotrophic lateral sclerosis, dementia, and other progressive degenerative diseases. Nonspecific indicators—such as progressive weight loss, a decline in plasma protein levels, and functional loss—are also used.

3.3 Heart Disease

In the USA, 58% of deaths are caused primarily or secondarily by cardiovascular disease [2]. The most characteristic cardiovascular death is death from cardiac arrest.

Patients with heart failure represent an additional challenge to the art of prognosis, since around 60% of them experience sudden cardiac death. The criteria for predicting cardiac arrest in these patients remain controversial [3, 4]. According to recent studies, prognostic factors include B-type natriuretic peptide (BNP), the ejection fraction, the end-diastolic diameter, the presence of nonsustained ventricular tachycardia, and the presence of diabetes mellitus [5, 6]. Precise evaluation of the incidence of cardiac arrest has become more complex because of the increased prevalence of automated implantable cardioverter–defibrillator use [7, 8].

The persistence of uncertainty about a patient's prognosis makes discussing their care preferences with them a very difficult moment, even in the best-case scenario. Findings from a study that involved cancer patients suggest that even a 10% chance of not surviving the next 6 months leads patients to ponder different treatment options [9]. It has been suggested that partly because of the uncertainty of their prognosis, patients who die from heart failure are those with the least understanding of their condition and the least involvement in the process of making decisions related to their care [11].

Table 3.3 Palliative Performance Scale (PPSv2): version 2

Level (%)	Ambulation	Activity and evidence of disease	Self-care	Intake	Conscious level
100	Full	Normal activity and work No evidence of disease	Full	Normal	Full
90	Full	Normal activity and work Some evidence of disease	Full	Normal	Full
80	Full	Normal activity with effort Some evidence of disease	Full	Normal or reduced	Full
70	Reduced	Unable normal job/work Significant disease	Full	Normal or reduced	Full
60	Reduced	Unable hobby/ housework Significant disease	Occasional assistance necessary	Normal or reduced	Full or confusion
50	Mainly sit/lie	Unable to do any work Extensive disease	Considerable assistance required	Normal or reduced	Full or confusion
40	Mainly in bed	Unable to do most activity Extensive disease	Mainly assistance	Normal or reduced	Full or drowsy ± confusion
30	Totally bed bound	Unable to do any activity Extensive disease	Total care	Normal or reduced	Full or drowsy ± confusion
20	Totally bed bound	Unable to do any activity Extensive disease	Total care	Minimal to sips	Full or drowsy ± confusion
10	Totally bed bound	Unable to do any activity Extensive disease	Total care	Mouth care only	Drowsy or coma ± confusion
0	Death	–	–	–	–

Reproduced from Victoria Hospice Society

A study of 274 deaths (26% of which were due to cardiovascular disease) concluded that a few therapies had been suspended or stopped in 84% of the patients. However, only 35% of those patients had been able to participate in the decision-making process [12]. Sick patients who die from heart failure but do not experience cardiac arrest undergo a gradual deterioration process, though it may be interrupted by acute episodes that frequently increase the risk of cardiac arrest, and this makes it even harder to generate predictive models.

Chronic cardiovascular conditions cause patients great suffering. Death generally occurs in a hospital, and although this tendency might correspond to the preferences of the patient and their family, patients with cardiovascular disease are less represented among those who receive home assistance and palliative care. In 2000, it was reported that patients with cardiovascular disease accounted for around 20% of all referrals to exclusive palliative care, whereas a 1996 study found that patients with cancer constituted more than 70% of users of American hospices [10]. It has been estimated that only 4% of patients with heart failure receive palliative care [7].

Uncertainty around predicting the trajectory of life's final stages in patients with heart failure may lead to what one article called "prognostic paralysis" concerning the beginning of the debate about palliative care and its effectiveness in cardiology [13]. One of the authors of the same article suggested that patients with heart failure should be considered candidates for palliative care if a physician were to answer "no" to the question "Would I be surprised if this patient died in the next 12 months?" [14]. In fact, this question is applicable in any critical clinical condition and could be considered the best criterion for recommending palliative care. The suggested 12-month period is very restricted if we think of the duration of life, but it is unbearably long if it corresponds to the duration of suffering.

Another suggested algorithm would initiate palliative care during or just after recovery from an acute exacerbation of heart failure. What seems clear from the experience of many services is that palliative care needs to be considered much earlier in the course of the cardiovascular disease process. The mark of these patients' suffering is shortness of breath.

3.4 Pulmonary Disease

As in most chronic illnesses, determining the prognosis or the life expectancy of patients with COPD is a subject filled with uncertainty. In all groups, age, smoking, decreased pulmonary function, and a low body mass index (BMI) are important mortality predictors [15–20]. Mortality predictors for elderly patients with COPD include the forced expiratory volume in 1 second (FEV_1), the gravity of physical disability, advanced age, and long-term use of oxygen, whereas use of tobacco, depression, quality of life, the presence of comorbidities, and the frequency of hospital admissions do not seem to predict mortality [21].

The frequency of COPD exacerbations, especially those that result in hospitalization, is correlated with increased mortality and is an independent predictor of a poor prognosis [22]. One study found that in patients aged 65 years or more, mortality rates following admission to an intensive care unit (ICU) during hospitalization for COPD exacerbation were high, reaching 30% during hospitalization and 59% within 1 year [23]. The same study showed that in-hospital and long-term mortality were strongly correlated with compromise of other organs and increased severity of pulmonary disease without a need for mechanical ventilation [23].

In the evolution of hospitalization due to a COPD exacerbation, the presence of comorbidities, a low quality-of-life index, major depression, and marital status have been shown to be strong predictors of mortality in elderly patients with COPD [24].

Even with many mortality predictors, it can be difficult to identify when a patient with COPD may be entering the final stage of their disease's evolution. Most of the usual COPD treatments are symptom related and of low toxicity. These factors limit the usefulness of a clear distinction between active disease treatment and palliative treatment, mainly in patients who experience periods of relative stability.

Around 20–25% of patients who present with severe COPD experience pain, depression, anxiety, and severe dyspnea at the end of their lives [25–27]. The intervention of palliative care may offer an opportunity for discussion about important aspects of end-of-life choices, such as knowing whether the patient will refuse intubation and mechanical ventilation, or would prefer to limit the duration of these interventions, accepting less invasive treatment options or even refusing hospitalization altogether.

Patients with advanced COPD are less likely to be moved to hospices than patients with lung cancer, even though the opportunities for discussion and choices concerning invasive ventilation support are rarer in patients with COPD [25].

3.5 Kidney Disease

It is known that nearly 20% of patients with kidney failure undergoing dialysis treatment stop dialysis before death. Almost all nephrologists are probably involved in end-of-life care of these patients with end-stage kidney disease (ESKD) [28]. However, doctors receive too little training or inadequate training in palliative care and are often uncomfortable with the care of dying patients [29, 30]. In a study involving American and Canadian doctors, for instance, only around 40% of 360 interviewed nephrologists affirmed that they were very well prepared for their patients' end-of-life decisions [30].

With the progression of kidney disease, palliative care becomes of greater importance and leads to more adequate symptom control and discussion regarding advanced directions, such as considering the possibility of discontinuing dialysis treatment if that is what the patient and their family choose. A UK paper on palliative care showed, yet again, opportunities to improve this aspect of ESKD care and led the authors to provide directions for palliative care [31].

3.6 Liver Disease

In the USA, chronic liver disease necessitates more than 1 million medical visits and more than 300,000 hospital admissions per year [32]. The evolution of liver disease causes patients to experience medical complications such as encephalopathy, malnutrition, muscle loss, ascites, esophagogastric variceal hemorrhage, spontaneous bacterial peritonitis, fatigue, and depression. Liver transplant—a valid treatment option—increases life expectancy and reduces many symptoms, but with the prevailing organ shortage, 10–15% of these patients die without receiving an organ. Many patients are also not transplant candidates, because of the presence of comorbidities. Moreover, some transplanted patients perish from complications of the transplant itself. Such patients and their families face the dilemma of a disease that is potentially treatable but still frequently fatal [32]. The initiation of palliative care in these patients proposes to offer them control of their symptoms, both while they are waiting for a transplant and also during their care after the procedure. The most intense interface presents itself in the condition of transplant rejection or detection of morbid conditions that aggravate the patient's clinical picture, such as liver cancer. The introduction of palliative care observes the commitment to maximize quality of life and, if possible, life expectancy.

3.7 Indications for Palliative Care in Intensive Care Units

Intensive care units (ICUs) provide sophisticated treatment for severely ill patients. Patients with chronic disease who experience exacerbations in their disease's evolution are living longer because of the advancements offered by their treatments—but generally with a worse quality of life. Unfortunately, there are still many obstacles in providing effective palliative care in health care, but—thanks to good medical practice based on evidence and common sense—science is on the side of palliative care [33]. In 2006, the journal *Critical Care Medicine* published a supplement dedicated to the theme of palliative care in the ICU, contemplating many dilemmas experienced in this area [31]. In a study presented at an American Thoracic Society conference in 2003, the researcher Judith Nelson reported that these obstacles include [32, 33]:

1. Insufficient communication concerning end-of-life decisions
2. Patient inability to participate in discussions concerning their treatment
3. Unrealistic expectations on the part of patients and their families about the prognosis or the efficacy of ICU treatment
4. Lack of opportunities for discussing the way that patients would like to receive end-of-life care

We may consider some situations found in intensive care that help us identify patients who could benefit from receiving attention from palliative care, nevertheless being in an intensive care environment (Tables 3.4 and 3.5).

3.8 HIV/AIDS

Despite advances in treatment of human immunodeficiency virus/acquired immunodeficiency syndrome (HIV/AIDS), there is still no known cure: the final result is always death. In contrast to other terminal illnesses such as cancer, it is not easy to

Table 3.4 Indications for palliative care in an intensive care unit [34]

Indication
Admission from a long-stay institution with one or more chronic limiting conditions (for example, dementia)
Two or more intensive care unit admissions in the same hospital
Prolonged time of mechanical ventilation mechanical ventilation or a failed attempt at weaning
Multiple organ failure
Candidacy for withdrawal of ventilatory support with the possibility of death
Metastatic cancer
Anoxic encephalopathy
Family suffering that prompts decision making

Table 3.5 Palliative care indications for patients with amyotrophic lateral sclerosis

Indication
A. Respiratory capacity decreased according to the following criteria:
1. Vital capacity <30% of normal
2. Significant dyspnea at rest
3. Need for supplemental oxygen at rest
4. Patient refuses artificial ventilation
B. Other indications for palliative care:
1. Progression to dependency and wheelchair ambulation
2. Difficulty speaking: speech that is poorly intelligible or unintelligible
3. Progression from normal diet to pureed diet
4. Progression of dependence in most or all major activities of daily living or need for assistance in all such activities
C. Critical nutritional compromise:
1. Intake of insufficient nutrients and fluids to sustain life
2. Continued weight loss
3. Dehydration or hypovolemia
4. Absence of artificial feeding methods
D. Life-threatening complications:
1. Recurrent aspiration pneumonia
2. Upper urinary tract infection
3. Sepsis
4. Recurrent fever after antibiotic therapy

predict when death is imminent. A patient with AIDS can die as a consequence of their first HIV manifestation or can be at constant risk of acquiring new diseases that may shorten their life. Most patients, however, will experience increasingly frequent health problems, ultimately reaching a stage of severe immunosuppression during a period of many years. As the disease progresses, treatment for symptomatic relief becomes more important than curative treatment.

Patients with AIDS are considered to be at the final stages of their disease if they have either of the following [1]:

1. CD4+ cell count ≤50% cells/μL
2. Persistent viral load >100,000 copies/mL

In association with any of the following:

1. Primary central nervous system (CNS) lymphoma
2. Loss of ≥33% of lean body mass
3. *Mycobacterium avium* bacteremia (untreated, not responding to treatment, or treatment refused)
4. Progressive multifocal leukoencephalopathy
5. Systemic lymphoma, with the disease being advanced by HIV and a partial response to chemotherapy
6. Therapy-insensitive visceral Kaposi's sarcoma
7. Kidney failure in the absence of dialysis
8. Cryptosporidiosis
9. Therapy-insensitive toxoplasmosis
10. Low performance status (≤50% on the Karnofsky Performance Status Scale)

AIDS patients must be referred to palliative care in the following scenarios [1]:

1. Persistent diarrhea for ≥1 year
2. Serum albumin level <2.5 g/dL
3. Persistent use of illegal drugs
4. Age >50 years
5. Absence of antiretroviral therapy, chemotherapy, and other medication associated with HIV disease prophylactics
6. Advanced HIV-associated dementia
7. Toxoplasmosis and symptomatic congestive heart failure at rest

3.9 Long-Term Neurological Disorders

Caring for high-risk patients with irreversible and progressive illness poses a daily challenge in the practice of palliative care. However, caring for patients who have serious, incurable illnesses that are progressing slowly and unpredictably, and whose need for assistance will irreversibly increase over time is still the greatest challenge for any health care professional.

Patients who have neurological disorders, whether they are of early onset or acquired at the last stage of life, experience low- or high-intensity physical, emotional, family, social, and spiritual suffering, but it frequently goes undetected by their doctors, caregivers, or relatives. The place for nononcological palliative care is being progressively recognized [35–38], especially in rapidly fatal neurological conditions such as motor neuron disease (MND) [37, 39], with many guidelines now recommending early referral to palliative care [40, 41]. These patients have different needs from those of cancer patients [36, 41, 42] and could be characterized as patients who experience symptoms of discomfort that are related to their neurological condition and highly variable in duration and intensity. Because of these patients' cognitive compromise, their symptoms are often evaluated indirectly through the perceptions of family or caregivers. With respect to palliative care, the following factors present difficulties in adequate handling of symptom management:

1. In general, neurological conditions evolve over a long course, and the onset of the disease's final stage is rarely clearly identifiable.
2. Symptoms may vary, and many of these patients have cognitive, behavioral, or communication disorders in addition to physical disabilities.

In this reality, it is very difficult to evaluate the difference between dysphasia and cognitive deficit, leading the palliative care team to require constant updates and training in the handling of these patients. Many physicians believe that rehabilitation is a short-term intervention related to a specific event. However, the handling of a chronic dysfunctional condition is a key factor in the success of the care provided to these patients, determining the quality of their end-of-life care [43, 44]. In the treatment of long-term neurological disorders, the interface between the neurologist, the physiatrist, and palliative care greatly clarifies their respective roles in the care of these patients and may be extended to other clinical conditions. It can also facilitate the liaison between the services that provide care (health care, insurance, and public services.)

A renowned British institution, the Royal College of Physicians, has published excellent care guidelines for patients with long-term neurological disorders [44]. Two of their goals were to explore the interaction between branches of medicine and to define the role of each in the care of patients under such conditions. Research has shown an alignment in the contributions made by each branch. The neurologist is involved in the evaluation, diagnosis, and management of the neurological condition. The physiatrist manages the patient's therapy, equipment, and social and psychological support during the phase between diagnosis and death. Specialists in palliative care are responsible for terminal care, handling the process of dying and grief.

3.10 Mental Illness

People with mental illness die prematurely in comparison with the general population. Despite the higher mortality rates among patients with mental illness, there have not been many reports or investigative studies concerning the planning of end-of-life care for these patients. Even basic information regarding the circumstances of death, health care preferences, and the availability of hospice and palliative care have never been evaluated for this population, not even in developed countries. This information is important for reasonable planning of practices, procedures, and guidelines aiming to offer quality end-of-life care for people with mental illness.

3.11 Stroke

The main criteria for palliative care referral of patients who have a cerebrovascular accident comprise nutritional status and functional capacity evaluation:

1. Palliative Performance Scale score (Table 3.3) ≤40%
2. Ambulation level: mainly in bed
3. Activity and evidence of disease: unable to do any activity
4. Incapacity for self-care
5. Diminished food and fluid intake
6. Consciousness level: drowsy/confused
7. Loss of >10% of body weight within the previous 6 months or >7.5% within the previous 3 months
8. Serum albumin level <2.5 g/dL
9. Current history of pulmonary aspiration with no effective response to interventions by a speech–language pathologist

3.12 Dementia

For patients with Alzheimer's disease and related conditions, the identification of certain structural alterations and functional compromise must serve as the basis for interventions and palliative care planning. The structural and functional disabilities associated with a primary diagnosis of Alzheimer's disease are often complicated by the presence of other comorbidities.

Ultimately, the combined effects of Alzheimer's disease (Functional Assessment Staging Test (FAST) stage 7) [45] and any other state of comorbidity or secondary condition (such as delirium, pressure ulcers, or aspiration pneumonia) must be such that a patient with Alzheimer's disease or a similar condition has a prognosis of ≤6 months' survival [1].

3.13 Amyotrophic Lateral Sclerosis

Amyotrophic lateral sclerosis (ALS) is a neurodegenerative disorder of unknown origin. It is progressive and causes death within an average of 3 or 4 years. Its incidence is estimated to be 1–2.5 cases per 100,000 people per year, with a prevalence of 2.5–8.5 cases per 100,000 people.

ALS tends to progress in a linear fashion over time, and so the overall functional decline in each patient is fairly constant and predictable. Although it generally manifests initially in one part of the body, the site of its initial manifestation does not determine the patient's life expectancy.

At the final stage of ALS, two factors are crucial for determining prognosis: the ability to breathe and, to a lesser extent, the ability to swallow [1].

Table 3.5 lists the indications for palliative care in patients with ALS. The patient is considered to be at the final stage of ALS if any of these indications have presented within the past 12 months.

3.14 Special Considerations

Some senior patients have a condition of severe frailty with no specific diagnosis but seem to have a progressive decline in vitality and appear to develop a predictable trajectory toward death within the following months.

For these patients, referral to palliative care is important in the sense of achieving the condition of global well-being. Unconventional palliative care referrals include referrals of elderly people with a progressive functional decline and progressive weight loss, and they may have multiple concurrent chronic conditions (for instance, high blood pressure, coronary artery disease, and diabetes) but no imminently fatal condition.

They may have had a recent advance in their cognitive and functional decline, or they may have made a decision not to proceed with aggressive treatment, because of their advanced age, general poor health, or poor cognitive state—or because of the excessive costs of such treatment.

For elderly patients, who are most vulnerable to these conditions, unexplained loss of ≥10% of body weight within a 6-month period or a BMI <22 kg/m^2 warrant palliative care.

Patients of all ages with a BMI <20 kg/m^2 who are sick enough to be hospitalized, independently of their diagnoses, have the highest mortality rate within 6 months after discharge.

The combination of progressive weight loss and difficulties in activities of daily living (ADLs) is an important predictor of mortality within 6 months—generally more important than the diagnosis, mental state, or ICU admission [1]. If these predictors are present, adequate communication with these patients and their families can establish a prospective management plan to reduce the stress caused by the worsening of these processes.

References

1. Christakis NA, Lamont EB. Extent and determinants of error in doctors' prognoses in terminally ill patients: prospective cohort study. BMJ. 2000;320(7233):469–72. https://doi.org/10.1136/bmj.320.7233.469.
2. Thom T, Haase N, Rosamond W, et al. Heart disease and stroke statistics—2006 update: a report from the American Heart Association Statistics Committee and Stroke Statistics Subcommittee. Circulation. 2006;113(6):e85–151. https://doi.org/10.1161/CIRCULATIONAHA.105.171600. Errata in: Circulation. 2006; 113 (14): e696 and Circulation. 2006; 114 (23): e630.
3. Maisel A. B-type natriuretic peptide levels: diagnostic and prognostic in congestive heart failure: what's next? Circulation. 2002;105(20):2328–31. https://doi.org/10.1161/01.cir.0000019121.91548.c2.
4. Berger R, Huelsman M, Strecker K, Bojic A, Moser P, Stanek B, Pacher R. B-type natriuretic peptide predicts sudden death in patients with chronic heart failure. Circulation. 2002;105(20):2392–7. https://doi.org/10.1161/01.cir.0000016642.15031.34.
5. Watanabe J, Shinozaki T, Shiba N, Fukahori K, Koseki Y, Karibe A, Sakuma M, Miura M, Kagaya Y, Shirato K. Accumulation of risk markers predicts the incidence of sudden

death in patients with chronic heart failure. Eur J Heart Fail. 2006;8(3):237–42. https://doi.org/10.1016/j.ejheart.2005.08.003.
6. Bardy GH, Lee KL, Mark DB, Poole JE, Packer DL, Boineau R, Domanski M, Troutman C, Anderson J, Johnson G, McNulty SE, Clapp-Channing N, Davidson-Ray LD, Fraulo ES, Fishbein DP, Luceri RM, Ip JH, Sudden Cardiac Death in Heart Failure Trial (SCD-HeFT) Investigators. Amiodarone or an implantable cardioverter–defibrillator for congestive heart failure. N Engl J Med. 2005;352(3):225–37. https://doi.org/10.1056/NEJMoa043399. Erratum in: N Engl J Med. 2005; 352 (20): 2146.
7. Daubert JP, Zareba W, Hall WJ, Schuger C, Corsello A, Leon AR, Andrews ML, McNitt S, Huang DT, Moss AJ, Study Investigators MADIT II. Predictive value of ventricular arrhythmia inducibility for subsequent ventricular tachycardia or ventricular fibrillation in Multicenter Automatic Defibrillator Implantation Trial (MADIT) II patients. J Am Coll Cardiol. 2006;47(1):98–107. https://doi.org/10.1016/j.jacc.2005.08.049.
8. Weeks JC, Cook EF, O'Day SJ, Peterson LM, Wenger N, Reding D, Harrell FE, Kussin P, Dawson NV, Connors AF Jr, Lynn J, Phillips RS. Relationship between cancer patients' predictions of prognosis and their treatment preferences. JAMA. 1998;279(21):1709–14. https://doi.org/10.1001/jama.279.21.1709. Erratum in: JAMA. 2000; 283 (2): 203.
9. Bouvy ML, Heerdink ER, Leufkens HG, Hoes AW. Predicting mortality in patients with heart failure: a pragmatic approach. Heart. 2003;89(6):605–9. https://doi.org/10.1136/heart.89.6.605.
10. Murray SA, Boyd K, Kendall M, Worth A, Benton TF, Clausen H. Dying of lung cancer or cardiac failure: prospective qualitative interview study of patients and their carers in the community. BMJ. 2002;325(7370):929. https://doi.org/10.1136/bmj.325.7370.929.
11. Faber-Langendoen K. A multi-institutional study of care given to patients dying in hospitals: ethical and practice implications. Arch Intern Med. 1996;156(18):2130–6.
12. Stewart S, McMurray JJ. Palliative care for heart failure. BMJ. 2002;325(7370):915–6. https://doi.org/10.1136/bmj.325.7370.915.
13. Murray SA, Boyd K, Sheikh A. Palliative care in chronic illness. BMJ. 2005;330(7492):611–2. https://doi.org/10.1136/bmj.330.7492.611.
14. Hauptman PJ, Havranek EP. Integrating palliative care into heart failure care. Arch Intern Med. 2005;165(4):374–8. https://doi.org/10.1001/archinte.165.4.374.
15. Landbo C, Prescott E, Lange P, Vestbo J, Almdal TP. Prognostic value of nutritional status in chronic obstructive pulmonary disease. Am J Respir Crit Care Med. 1999;160(6):1856 61. https://doi.org/10.1164/ajrccm.160.6.9902115.
16. Anthonisen NR, Wright EC, Hodgkin JE. Prognosis in chronic obstructive pulmonary disease. Am Rev Respir Dis. 1986;133(1):14–20. https://doi.org/10.1164/arrd.1986.133.1.14.
17. Kanner RE, Renzetti AD Jr, Stanish WM, Barkman HW Jr, Klauber MR. Predictors of survival in subjects with chronic airflow limitation. Am J Med. 1983;74(2).249–55. https://doi.org/10.1016/0002-9343(83)90623-x.
18. Postma DS, Gimeno F, van der Weele LT, Sluiter HJ. Assessment of ventilatory variables in survival prediction of patients with chronic airflow obstruction: the importance of reversibility. Eur J Respir Dis. 1985;67(5):360–8.
19. Burrows B, Earle RH. Prediction of survival in patients with chronic airway obstruction. Am Rev Respir Dis. 1969;99(6):865–71. https://doi.org/10.1164/arrd.1969.99.6.865.
20. Yohannes AM, Baldwin RC, Connolly M. Mortality predictors in disabling chronic obstructive pulmonary disease in old age. Age Ageing. 2002;31(2):137–40. https://doi.org/10.1093/ageing/31.2.137.
21. Soler-Cataluña JJ, Martínez-García MA, Román Sánchez P, Salcedo E, Navarro M, Ochando R. Severe acute exacerbations and mortality in patients with chronic obstructive pulmonary disease. Thorax. 2005;60(11):925–31. https://doi.org/10.1136/thx.2005.040527.
22. Seneff MG, Wagner DP, Wagner RP, Zimmerman JE, Knaus WA. Hospital and 1-year survival of patients admitted to intensive care units with acute exacerbation of chronic obstructive pulmonary disease. JAMA. 1995;274(23):1852–7.

23. Almagro P, Calbo E, Ochoa de Echagüen A, Barreiro B, Quintana S, Heredia JL, Garau J. Mortality after hospitalization for COPD. Chest. 2002;121(5):1441–8. https://doi.org/10.1378/chest.121.5.1441.
24. Claessens MT, Lynn J, Zhong Z, Desbiens NA, Phillips RS, Wu AW, Harrell FE Jr, Connors AF Jr. Dying with lung cancer or chronic obstructive pulmonary disease: insights from SUPPORT. Study to Understand Prognoses and Preferences for Outcomes and Risks of Treatments. J Am Geriatr Soc. 2000;48(S1):S146–53. https://doi.org/10.1111/j.1532-5415.2000.tb03124.x.
25. Lynn J, Ely EW, Zhong Z, McNiff KL, Dawson NV, Connors A, Desbiens NA, Claessens M, McCarthy EP. Living and dying with chronic obstructive pulmonary disease. J Am Geriatr Soc. 2000;48(S1):S91–S100. https://doi.org/10.1111/j.1532-5415.2000.tb03147.x.
26. Elkington H, White P, Addington-Hall J, Higgs R, Pettinari C. The last year of life of COPD: a qualitative study of symptoms and services. Respir Med. 2004;98(5):439–45. https://doi.org/10.1016/j.rmed.2003.11.006.
27. Holley JL. Palliative care for patients with end-stage kidney disease: UpToDate. https://www.uptodate.com/contents/palliative-care-for-patients-with-end-stage-kidney-disease. Accessed
28. Holley JL, Carmody SS, Moss AH, Sullivan AM, Cohen LM, Block SD, Arnold RM. The need for end-of-life care training in nephrology: national survey results of nephrology fellows. Am J Kidney Dis. 2003;42(4):813–20. https://doi.org/10.1016/s0272-6386(03)00868-0.
29. Davison SN, Jhangri GS, Holley JL, Moss AH. Nephrologists' reported preparedness for end-of-life decision-making. Clin J Am Soc Nephrol. 2006;1(6):1256–62. https://doi.org/10.2215/CJN.02040606.
30. Gunda S, Thomas M, Smith S. National survey of palliative care in end-stage renal disease in the UK. Nephrol Dial Transplant. 2005;20(2):392–5. https://doi.org/10.1093/ndt/gfh619.
31. Larson AM, Curtis JR. Integrating palliative care for liver transplant candidates: "too well for transplant, too sick for life". JAMA. 2006;295(18):2168–76. https://doi.org/10.1001/jama.295.18.2168.
32. Farmer JC, Levy MM, Curtis JR. Improving the quality of end-of-life care in the ICU. Crit Care Med. 2006;34(11 Suppl):S301–420. https://journals.lww.com/ccmjournal/toc/2006/11001#1047571941. Accessed 10 Aug 2020.
33. Nelson JE, Meier DE. Palliative care in the intensive care unit: part I. J Intensive Care Med. 1999;14(4):130–9. https://doi.org/10.1046/j.1525-1489.1998.00130.x.
34. Nelson JE, Danis M. End-of-life care in the intensive care unit: where are we now? Crit Care Med. 2001;29(2 Suppl):N2–9. https://doi.org/10.1097/00003246-200102001-00002.
35. O'Brien T. Neurodegenerative disease. In: Addington-Hall JM, Higgonson IJ, editors. Palliative care for non-cancer patients. Oxford: Oxford University Press; 2001. p. 44–53.
36. Murtagh FE, Preston M, Higginson I. Patterns of dying: palliative care for non-malignant disease. Clin Med (Lond). 2004;4(1):39–44. https://doi.org/10.7861/clinmedicine.4-1-39.
37. Royal College of Physicians. Palliative care services: meeting the needs of patients. In: Report of a working party 2007. London: Royal College of Physicians; 2007. https://shop.rcplondon.ac.uk/products/palliative-care-services-meeting-the-needs-of-patients?variant=6634703045. Accessed 10 Aug 2020.
38. O'Brien T, Kelly M, Saunders C. Motor neurone disease: a hospice perspective. BMJ. 1992;304(6825):471–3. https://doi.org/10.1136/bmj.304.6825.471.
39. National Collaborating Centre for Chronic Conditions. Multiple sclerosis: national clinical guidelines for diagnosis and management in primary and secondary care. London: Royal College of Physicians; 2004.
40. National Institute for Clinical Excellence. Guidance on cancer services: improving supportive and palliative care for adults with cancer: the manual. London: National Institute for Clinical Excellence; 2004. https://www.nice.org.uk/guidance/csg4/resources/improving-supportive-and-palliative-care-for-adults-with-cancer-pdf-773375005. Accessed 10 Aug 2020.
41. Voltz R, Borasio GD. Palliative therapy in the terminal stage of neurological disease. J Neurol. 1997;244(Suppl 4):S2–S10. https://doi.org/10.1007/PL00007721.

42. Miller RG, Rosenberg JA, Gelinas DF, Mitsumoto H, Newman D, Sufit R, Borasio GD, Bradley WG, Bromberg MB, Brooks BR, Kasarskis EJ, Munsat TL. Oppenheimer EA; the ALS Practice Parameters Task Force. Practice parameter: the care of the patient with amyotrophic lateral sclerosis (an evidence-based review): report of the Quality Standards Subcommittee of the American Academy of Neurology: ALS Practice Parameters Task Force. Neurology. 1999;52(7):1311–23. https://doi.org/10.1212/wnl.52.7.1311.
43. Johnson J, Smith P, Goldstone L. Executive summary. In: Johnson J, Smith P, Goldstone L, editors. Evaluation of MS specialist nurses: a review and development of the role. Letchworth Garden City: MS Research Trust; 2001. p. 8–25. https://www.mstrust.org.uk/sites/default/files/files/Johnson et al Evaluation of MS Specialist Nurses.pdf. Accessed 10 Aug 2020.
44. Royal College of Physicians, National Council for Palliative Care, British Society of Rehabilitation Medicine. Long-term neurological conditions: management at the interface between neurology, rehabilitation and palliative care. London: Royal College of Physicians; 2008. https://www.rcplondon.ac.uk/guidelines-policy/long-term-neurological-conditions. Accessed 10 Aug 2020.
45. Reisberg B. Functional assessment staging (FAST). Psychopharmacol Bull. 1998;24(4):653–9.

Chapter 4
Evaluation of Suffering in Adults and the Elderly

"To grow old and die" is not on the list of the best experiences that we can have in most countries. With the advances of the Industrial Revolution and its educational, scientific, and technological developments, it became clear that economic development has two effects on the population: (1) it reduces mortality rates in general, reduces infant mortality in particular, and makes it possible to increase the population's living conditions; and (2) after a certain period of time when mortality starts to fall, fertility rates also start to fall, causing a decrease in the size of families.

At first, there was an increase in population growth rates, but with the drop in birth rates, the population growth rate decreased, tending toward stability. This phenomenon, typical of the twentieth century, is called demographic transition (DT). An unequivocal gain was that the average life expectancy of the world's population doubled within a century, increasing from around 30 years in 1900 to more than 60 years in 2000. First, let us look at the aging horizon in the world [1]. In 1986, the demographers Ron Lesthaeghe and Dirk Van de Kaa wrote a text that spoke, for the first time, of the second demographic transition (SDT) [2]. In 1987, Van de Kaa described the main characteristics of the SDT in Europe (Table 4.1).

Table 4.1 The main characteristics of the second demographic transition in Europe [2]

Characteristic
Fertility rates below the replacement level
Postponement of the birth of the first child
Growth in the number of children born outside of marriage
Change in the patterns of marriage and maternity/paternity
Growth of cohabitation and consensual unions
Diversification of family and home arrangements
Growth in the numbers of divorces and separations
Change in focus from families with children to adult couples (changing the direction of the intergenerational flow of wealth)
Growth in immigration

A. C. L. Q. Arantes, *Clinical Assessment of Human Suffering*,
https://doi.org/10.1007/978-3-030-57535-9_4

In 2006, Coleman wrote an article considering the definitions of the third demographic transition that has affected Europe and the USA [3]. The ancestral characteristics of some populations are being radically altered by immigration of large numbers of people from distant geographical regions in combination with insufficient fertility rates for population replacement and emigration of domestic savings.

The *World Population Prospects 2019* review [4, 5] is the 26th edition of the United Nations' population estimates and projections. It presents population estimates from 1950 to the present for 235 countries or areas, supported by analyses of historical demographic trends. This last evaluation considers the results of 1690 national population censuses carried out between 1950 and 2018, in addition to information from registries and 2700 representative national sample surveys. The 2019 review also presents population projections for the year 2100 that reflect a series of plausible results at the global, regional, and national levels.

Since the 1950s, most elderly people have lived in Third World countries—a fact that has not yet been appreciated by many who continue to associate old age with the more developed countries in Europe or North America. In fact, as early as 1960, more than half of all people aged ≥65 years lived in Third World countries. In Latin America, it was predicted that between 1980 and 2000, a 120% increase in the total population would occur (from 363.7 million to 803.6 million), while the increase in the population over 60 years of age would be 236% (from 23.3 million to 78.2 million)—that is, twice as great as the percentage increase in the population as a whole [6]. In the longer term, the outlook was even more dramatic.

Now we take a closer look at the world of the person who ages under a physiological process that is hidden from the vast majority of health professionals.

The biological context of aging and appropriate management of multiple concurrent diseases—added to the whole challenge of managing relational models in transformation and the delicate family context and personal nucleus of an elderly person who needs to face the progressive loss of autonomy and independence that accompany aging in our world (Fig. 4.1)—also form the basis for the knowledge and practice of every geriatrician and gerontologist with recognized training. According to projections from the United Nations Population Fund, one in nine

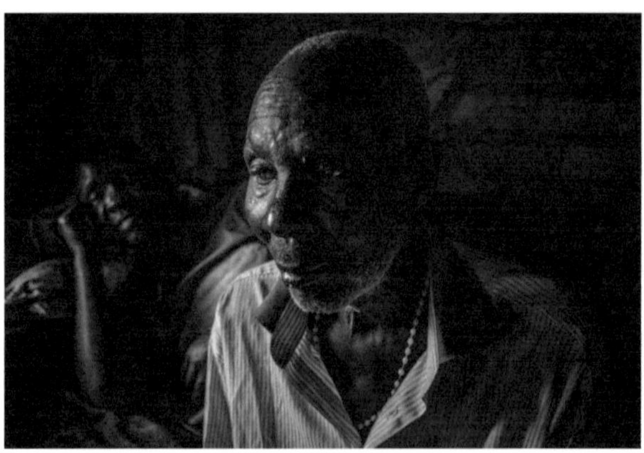

Fig. 4.1 The elderly person must face progressive losses

people in the world is aged 60 years or more, and this proportion is estimated to grow to one in five by 2050.

Studies show that inappropriate prescribing is an important and possibly preventable risk factor for adverse reactions to medications in the elderly, and hospital-based studies have shown that a large proportion of hospitalizations are the result of these reactions. The most common conclusion of these studies is that use of multiple medications prescribed by different specialists who are treating an elderly patient concurrently is common and that inappropriate use of medications is associated with acute hospitalization in elderly people living in the community. These results indicate that it is desirable, with the current knowledge, to reduce these complications through provision of appropriate information to doctors and more careful prescribing [7].

It seems rather obvious that major medical advances could not have happened without the generosity of young and old clinical trial participants. It is very important for clinical studies to include participants of different ages, sexes, races, and ethnicities. When clinical research involves a group of people who are similar, the findings may not be applicable to or beneficial for everyone. The paradox we are experiencing today is that the elderly are the major users of many medicines. Literature data show that although people aged ≥65 years represent only about 13% of the population, they consume almost a third of all medicines.

The population of older patients is poorly represented in clinical trials, with up to 35% of published trials excluding the elderly [8]. Recently, it has been argued that the aging crisis should be addressed by developing broader expertise and research in geriatric pharmacology. The elderly have been found to be underrepresented in cancer clinical trials, and this finding was more pronounced in studies in early-stage cancer than in studies in advanced-stage cancer.

There is inadequate evidence and knowledge of geriatric patients' responses to medications. In the USA, although people aged ≥65 years account for 61% of all new cancer cases and 70% of all cancer deaths, in active oncological clinical trials performed between 1993 and 1996, only 25% of participants in the studies were elderly [9]. One study in Ireland audited 226 clinical research proposals that were submitted for ethical approval, in order to ascertain how many of them excluded participants on the basis of an arbitrary upper age limit. It found that a significant proportion (13.7%) of the proposals did so, but among the relevant proposals that were submitted by geriatricians (9.8%), there were none that excluded participants on the basis of age alone. More than 50% of the proposals submitted in neurology/psychiatry did exclude participants on the basis of an upper age limit.

The elderly have well-known features of more chronic diseases and weaknesses, with fewer social and financial resources. Even in the absence of chronic disease, aging entails some loss of function. With so many adverse situations, care of the elderly needs to be structured differently from that of younger adults. The current provision of health services fragments care of the elderly, with multiplication of specialist consultations, lack of information sharing, and use of numerous drugs, clinical examinations, and imaging and other procedures. This systemic overload has major financial impacts at all levels without conferring significant benefits on health or quality of life [10].

There is evidence that care of the elderly needs to be organized in an integrated manner and coordinated through a care pathway—a logical network between the health system and end-of-life care [11]. Suitable models of health care for seniors are those with care pathways focused on education initiatives, health promotion, prevention of preventable diseases, early care, and rehabilitation [12]. In short, to be effective, a model of health care for the elderly must be applicable to the levels of care required; that is, it must have a well-designed flow of educational activities, health promotion, and prevention of preventable diseases. This care pathway starts with the initial engagement with the elderly person and their evaluation and monitoring, and should continue right up until the final moments of their life in a palliative care unit. So, to put in place all necessary actions for healthy aging and quality of life, we need to rethink and redesign the care of the elderly, focusing on the individual and their uniqueness.

4.1 Dying in the Twenty-First Century

In 1900, people had an average life expectancy of around 30 years because infant mortality was high and infections and wars were common causes of death. The average dependency time after the onset of major illness was short. However, in the year 2000, we passed an average life expectancy of more than 60 years, and cancer, cardiovascular disease, and dementia are now common causes of death. The average dependency time in elderly people is around 2–4 years. The suffering caused by this dependency time has five dimensions, each of which has its own impacts. Aging favors the appearance of diseases that are more prevalent in old age, and three major groups of diseases make this stage of life even more challenging: cancer, cardiovascular disease, and dementias.

Regarding dementia, we know that it is a syndrome caused by various diseases with a slow and progressive course, affecting memory, thinking, reasoning, orientation, understanding, learning ability, language, judgment, behavior, and the ability to perform activities of daily living, with varying durations (depending on their cause) ranging from 2 to 12 years. Dementia mainly affects the elderly, but it is estimated that 2–10% of all cases begin before the age of 65 years. After that age, the prevalence doubles every 5 years. Dementia is one of the main causes of dependence and disability in old age [13].

Regarding Alzheimer's disease, the expectation is that by 2050, 131.5 million people worldwide will be affected by this disease. The total number of new cases of dementia each year is almost 9.9 million worldwide, which means that a diagnosis of Alzheimer's disease is made every 3 seconds. These updated estimates are 15% higher for 2030 and 17% higher for 2050 than the previous estimates for those years recorded in the *World Alzheimer Report 2009* [14].

As yet, Alzheimer's disease has no cure. The highest risk factor for Alzheimer's disease is old age. Most diagnoses of Alzheimer's disease are made in people aged ≥65 years. The diagnosis of dementia is based on criteria listed in the 2013 edition of the American Psychiatric Association's *Diagnostic and Statistical Manual of Mental Disorders* (DSM-5) [15].

What is life, after all? A definition I favor is that life is a sexually transmitted, incurable, progressive condition, which can lead to several disabilities and which, in 100% of cases, leads to death; that is, absolutely all of us will die. In the time of dependency, in the Brazilian reality, we have elderly people taking care of other elderly people, or—more often than we would like to believe is the case—there is no one who cares.

And so goes our humanity. But being like this does not prevent us from experiencing all of the suffering within reach of a disease that comes without pity from our body, from our fears, from our loves. Disease arrives and threatens the continuity of life. No matter what the origin is of this human being who gets sick, suffering will make a home in his life and, if there is no way to mitigate all of this, the end will almost always be a misery.

Facing a disease that threatens the continuity of life is one of our most challenging encounters with our fragility, vulnerability, and helplessness.

Think about this difficult but important reflection: Suppose that in a year, illness and suffering will come to stay in your life for some time. How would you feel if someone you love was in pain or suffering from symptoms that the most advanced technologies could not manage? How would you feel if the doctor taking care of you did not know how to assess and/or treat your pain and suffering? What if you had no hope that your pain and suffering could be relieved?

The process of changing attitudes starts with training and with information so that people know what to do. It then goes through a stage of finding out how to do it. But behavioral change takes time until people who know what to do, and how to do it, actually do what needs to be done.

Although scientific advances in medicine have hijacked death and turned it into an almost taboo event that happens in a hospital, it needs to be returned to humanity [16]. We have the right to a dignified death, just as we are entitled to a decent life, regardless of our age. And although death is a big taboo, no one escapes without encountering this stage of life at some point—either when we ourselves are seriously ill or when we experience the death of someone very close to us. Death is an unforgettable experience when it is your own or that of someone you love. The dignity of life must be a right for all inhabitants of this world, and this experience of the dignity of human life can offer its best performance with good palliative care practice.

Death—to be a day worth living—needs care.

References

1. Alves JED, Cavenaghi SM. Population and development: the third demographic transition [in Portuguese]. Instituto de Economia da UFRJ. http://www.ie.ufrj.br/aparte/pdfs/ttd_aparte_16fev08.pdf. Accessed.

2. Van De Kaa DJ. Europe's second demographic transition. Popul Bull. 1987;42(1):1–59.
3. Coleman D. Immigration and ethnic change in low-fertility countries: a third demographic transition. Popul Dev Rev. 2006;32(3):401–66.
4. Population Division, United Nations Department of Economic and Social Affairs. World population prospects 2019: highlights. New York: United Nations; 2019. https://population.un.org/wpp/Publications/Files/WPP2019_Highlights.pdf. Accessed 10 Aug 2020.
5. Haub C, Gribble J. The world at 7 billion. Popul Bull. 2011;66(2). https://www.prb.org/wp-content/uploads/2011/07/world-at-7-billion.pdf. Accessed 10 Aug 2020.
6. Ramos LR, Veras RP, Kalache A. Envelhecimento populacional: uma realidade Brasileira [Population aging: a Brazilian reality]. Rev Saude Publica. 1987;21(3):211–24.
7. Stefano ICA, Conterno LO, da Silva Filho CR, Marin MJ. Uso de medicamentos por idosos: análise da prescrição, dispensação e utilização num município de porte médio do estado de São Paulo [Medication use by the elderly: analysis of prescribing, dispensing, and use in a medium-sized city in the state of Sao Paulo]. Revista Brasileira de Geriatria e Gerontologia. 2017;20(5):679–90. https://doi.org/10.1590/1981-22562017020.170062.
8. Secoli SR. Polifarmácia: interações e reações adversas no uso de medicamentos por idosos [Polypharmacy: interaction and adverse reactions in the use of drugs by elderly people]. Rev Bras Enferm. 2010;63(1):136–40. https://doi.org/10.1590/s0034-71672010000100023.
9. Shenoy P, Harugeri A. Elderly patients' participation in clinical trials. Perspect Clin Res. 2015;6(4):184-189. doi:10.4103/2229-3485.1670990. https://doi.org/10.4103/2229-3485.167099.
10. Silva VDL, Cesse EÂ, de Albuquerque MDF. Determinantes sociais da mortalidade do idoso: uma revisão sistemática da literatura [Social determinants of death among the elderly: a systematic literature review]. Rev Bras Epidemiol. 2014;17(Suppl 2):178–93. https://doi.org/10.1590/1809-4503201400060015.
11. Veras R, Oliveira M. Linha de cuidado para o idoso: detalhando o modelo [Care pathway for the elderly: detailing the model]. Revista Brasileira de Geriatria e Gerontologia. 2016;19(6):887–905.
12. Oliveira MR, Silveira DP, Neves R, Veras R, Estrella K, Assalim VM, Araujo DV, Gomes GHG, Lima KC. Idoso na saúde suplementar: uma urgência para a saúde da sociedade e para a sustentabilidade do setor [Elderly in supplementary health: an urgency for the health of society and for the sustainability of the sector]. Rio de Janeiro: National Supplementary Health Agency; 2016.
13. Burlá C, Camarano AA, Kanso S, Fernandes D, Nunes R. Panorama prospectivo das demências no Brasil: um enfoque demográfico [A perspective overview of dementia in Brazil: a demographic approach]. Cien Saude Colet. 2013;18(10):2949–56. https://doi.org/10.1590/s1413-81232013001000019.
14. Prince M, Jackson J, editors. World Alzheimer report 2009. London: Alzheimer's Disease International; 2009. https://www.alz.co.uk/research/files/WorldAlzheimerReport.pdf. Accessed.
15. American Psychiatric Association. Diagnostic and statistical manual of mental disorders. 5th ed. Washington, DC: American Psychiatric Association; 2013.
16. Arantes ACQ. A morte é um dia que vale a pena viver [Death is a day worth living]. 2nd ed. Sao Paulo: Sextante; 2019.

Chapter 5
How Good Conversations Can Be

When we think of difficult news, we need a very important initial parameter. Bad news is any information that has the power to change a person's future for the worse. Something bad has been reported, and that is why life can enter a very difficult time to be experienced. Another important aspect to know is that the doctor who communicates bad news is someone who suffers from having to do this. That is why you avoid this situation at all costs, and if you cannot escape this function by delegating it, you need a lot of guidance on how to do it. And here our challenge begins: most of us have received no technical guidance on how to proceed with this moment of the doctor–patient relationship—and certainly no guidance on how to do so humanely (Fig. 5.1).

I remember, with great regret, my "first time." In my first year of residency at a medical clinic, I attended a 17-year-old girl in the general medical teaching clinic. Her presenting complaints flowed into a somewhat dangerous diagnostic hypothesis: a viral process. On this occasion, the cruel presence of acquired

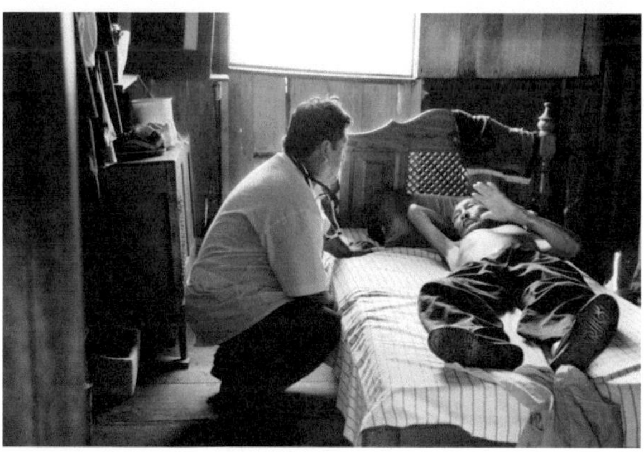

Fig. 5.1 The doctor–patient relationship is as important as the technical knowledge

A. C. L. Q. Arantes, *Clinical Assessment of Human Suffering*,
https://doi.org/10.1007/978-3-030-57535-9_5

immunodeficiency syndrome (AIDS) became very real as one of the possibilities, although the girl had no obvious risk behavior, no drug use, no history of transfusion, and a stable partner—a 19-year-old boyfriend to whom she hoped to become engaged within a year. During our conversation, I informed her about routine tests, including the test for human immunodeficiency virus (HIV). There was no semblance of concern about it; after all, it was a routine test for complaints, signs, and symptoms of her presenting condition. Three weeks later, her test results were returned. I opened the laboratory envelopes, already available inside the patient's chart: she was HIV positive, without any doubt, judging by the antibody levels recorded. I walked toward the assistants' room to discuss the case, visibly shaken by the diagnosis I had just made. One assistant's reaction was absurd: laughing out loud, he commented to his colleagues, "Now the doctor here will know what it's like to be a doctor!" I asked how I could possibly deliver this news. He replied that he should tell her and should do so in the presence of her mother or a guardian, as she was a minor.

"How do I do this?"

"Go out there and talk."

Go out there and talk.

That was the guidance I received from a medical clinic professor on how to deliver bad news. Most of my professional colleagues who did not receive guidance on how to deliver difficult news had to deal with the inability of our teachers to teach us something that I consider to be one of the most valuable and delicate aspects of the relationship between a doctor and their patient.

For a long time, I suffered from not knowing how to improve my conversational technique, but when I read Elisabeth Kübler Ross's book *On Death and Dying* [1] —a book that described her conversations with terminally ill cancer patients—I found that it can be easier to talk when we know how to give more importance to what is said, and who is listening, than to our insecurity about this moment.

In college, the first bad news that we received indirectly was that we would not receive adequate preparation for how to deal with our humanity in the face of the suffering of each patient we would go on to care for. The good news is that this reality is now changing, and the knowledge necessary for knowing how to talk about difficult news, and how to do it well, exists and is available to all who wish to obtain it.

For a good conversation, I think, the first step is to choose what will be covered by your attention. Do not focus on the subject of the disease, nor on the results of laboratory or imaging tests. We can use these resources, but only to inform and help us to be more aware of our role in the life of this person who needs our care and is listening carefully. First, look the patient in the eye. Maintain your attentive and loyal focus on the person who has the disease, and their perspective, and refocus your attention on what really matters. Looking into the patient's eyes, you realize that that person is much more than their illness. Looking into their eyes, you have an idea of the greatness of this human being. Sometimes, the extent of what we see is such that it is necessary to ask questions with a sense of urgency. But focus with full attention on not asking stifling questions. You need to learn to ask open-ended questions, as they have great power; they favor creation—not creation in the sense of inventing answers, but creation of a path specific to this person who, day by day, is living and building the path of this experience of their time to die, and that only happens when the question allows them to explore spaces within them that lead them to the answers that already inhabit them but have never been discovered. Knowing how to ask questions can be learned only by those who know how to look. Because they know how to look, they know how to ask. Looking expands our capacity to be curious in the face of an unknown reality—in this case, the reality of the experience that the patient has lived before their illness and all of the consequences (of the illness).

Look, ask—and listen. Listening in the way you would like to be heard is the only part of the illness experience that can be shared between the human being who cares and the one who receives that care. In the same way, the time they exchange with each other is exactly the same; if I give you 15 minutes of my time, I will have 15 minutes of your time for me. The account is mathematical. But, in terms of the content that fills this time, we speak of listening. I am heard, and I can hear. And these skills should be carefully trained so that our listening prevails over our speech, especially when it comes to taking care of people in their final time. The person who dies does not have time to waste on our need to speak, threaten, or exercise power over him. We are the ones who need to know how to listen. Do not listen with simultaneous thought of resolution or interpretation of what is being said. Listen with your whole body, with your soul, with your existence. Listen as if your life also depends on it. This person's life—the meaning of this life that you care for—may depend on your ability to hear what they have to say about what is important to them.

Then receive, as a gift, everything that has been said. The suffering that the patient shares with us is a gift. Feeling gratitude for this trust already leads us to a wider space of wisdom about caring. Sometimes it can be a heavy gift, well wrapped, buried in a lot of pain and fear. And our role will be to carry this gift, received in listening, to join our own treasures. Then it is time to look at our being, our humanity, our technical knowledge, our available resources, and, with each of these resources, open the gift delivered by the patient. We often want to help a person in these conditions, but, as we do not know what to do, we make the decision to put ourselves in their place to experience their suffering. This is empathy—a necessary step, no doubt—but it cannot balance us. Choosing to stop at empathy is like walking a tightrope and deciding to walk it on one foot. Balancing yourself only on the perception of suffering that does not belong to you is impossible to do for a long time. It leads to extreme emotional tiredness, the fatigue of empathy. That is why this moment is important—to receive this suffering, presented as a gift, and to separate out our tools to be able to open it. This is the greatest exercise in care. Respect the suffering of others, but also know in detail everything we have and are, in order to take care of this suffering.

Then act. Action is the basis for transforming reality. The action that happens from the awareness of one who embraces the role as a caregiver, from the consciousness of the suffering established by the patient as a care priority, listens attentively. A revolution happens when we become aware of everything we have and are, in order to practice care. Then act: act for the relief of suffering; act to provide patients and their families with the possibility of exercising happiness in their history.

Doctor–patient communication is widely considered an essential attribute of high-quality care [2]. In the end-of-life scenario, in particular, research and teaching efforts are focused on this specific aspect of the doctor–patient relationship [3–12]. But the doctor–patient relationship encompasses more than just communication. Patients whose lives are fully valued in their final time are seen as a whole person by their doctor [13, 14]; receive care from their personal doctor [14, 15]; have a doctor with whom fears can be discussed [14]; have a relationship based on mutual respect, trust, and humility [16]; and receive care that is attentive to their emotions [14, 15].

References

1. Kübler-Ross E. On death and dying. New York: Scribner; 1969.
2. Institute of Medicine Committee on Quality of Health Care in America. Crossing the quality chasm: a new health system for the 21st century. Washington, DC: National Academies Press; 2001.
3. Back AL, Arnold RM, Baile WF, Fryer-Edwards KA, Alexander SC, Barley GE, Gooley TA, Tulsky JA. Efficacy of communication skills training for giving bad news and discussing transitions to palliative care. Arch Intern Med. 2007;167(5):453–60. https://doi.org/10.1001/archinte.167.5.453.
4. Back AL, Arnold RM, Baile WF, Tulsky JA, Fryer-Edwards K. Approaching difficult communication tasks in oncology. CA Cancer J Clin. 2005;55(3):164–77. https://doi.org/10.3322/canjclin.55.3.164.
5. Sullivan AM, Lakoma MD, Billings JA, Peters AS, Block SD, PCEP Core Faculty. Creating enduring change: demonstrating the long-term impact of a faculty development program in palliative care. J Gen Intern Med. 2006;21(9):907–14. https://doi.org/10.1111/j.1525-1497.2006.00486.x.
6. Sullivan AM, Lakoma MD, Block SD. The status of medical education in end-of-life care: a national report. J Gen Intern Med. 2003;18(9):685–95. https://doi.org/10.1046/j.1525-1497.2003.21215.x.
7. Tulsky JA. Beyond advance directives: importance of communication skills at the end of life. JAMA. 2005;294(3):359–65. https://doi.org/10.1001/jama.294.3.359.
8. Butow PN, Dowsett S, Hagerty R, Tattersall MH. Communicating prognosis to patients with metastatic disease: what do they really want to know? Support Care Cancer. 2002;10(2):161–8. https://doi.org/10.1007/s005200100290.
9. Christakis NA, Iwashyna TJ. Attitude and self-reported practice regarding prognostication in a national sample of internists. Arch Intern Med. 1998;158(21):2389–95. https://doi.org/10.1001/archinte.158.21.2389.
10. Clayton JM, Butow PN, Arnold RM, Tattersall MH. Fostering coping and nurturing hope when discussing the future with terminally ill cancer patients and their caregivers. Cancer. 2005;103(9):1965–75. https://doi.org/10.1002/cncr.21011.
11. Weeks JC, Cook EF, O'Day SJ, et al. Relationship between cancer patients' predictions of prognosis and their treatment preferences. JAMA. 1998;279(21):1709–14. https://doi.org/10.1001/jama.279.21.1709. Erratum in: JAMA. 2000; 283 (2): 203.

12. Smith R. Patient-centered interview: an evidence-based method. Philadelphia: Lippincott Williams and Wilkins; 2002.
13. Steinhauser KE, Christakis NA, Clipp EC, McNeilly M, McIntyre L, Tulsky JA. Factors considered important at the end of life by patients, family, physicians, and other care providers. JAMA. 2000;284(19):2476–82. https://doi.org/10.1001/jama.284.19.2476.
14. Teno JM, Clarridge BR, Casey V, et al. Family perspectives on end-of-life care at the last place of care. JAMA. 2004;291(1):88–93. https://doi.org/10.1001/jama.291.1.88.
15. Wenrich MD, Curtis JR, Ambrozy DA, Carline JD, Shannon SE, Ramsey PG. Dying patients' need for emotional support and personalized care from physicians. perspectives of patients with terminal illness, families, and health care providers. J Pain Symptom Manage. 2003;25(3):236–46. https://doi.org/10.1016/s0885-3924(02)00694-2.
16. Curtis JR, Wenrich MD, Carline JD, Shannon SE, Ambrozy DM, Ramsey PG. Understanding physicians' skills at providing end-of-life care perspectives of patients, families, and health care workers. J Gen Intern Med. 2001;16(1):41–9. https://doi.org/10.1111/j.1525-1497.2001.00333.x.

Chapter 6
Dimensions of Care

6.1 The Biological Dimension

In the palliative care approach, the greatest will is the patient's, and their voice is the one that governs and determines the direction of care. Therefore, a well-conducted assessment is the first and most fundamental step toward the success of this work. An insufficient or imprecise evaluation can result in a succession of errors and mistakes in diagnostic or therapeutic procedures. And since a person's time is precious, especially at the end of their life, an error in approach bleeds important moments that can never return. We are multidimensional beings. We will never be just a body or a disease. We have our history and our biography, and in this biography we have our faces, composed of broad dimensions that characterize us:

1. The body, in its biological dimension—which makes us feel the internal world. When hearing a serious disease, the body starts to express signs and symptoms of discomfort, which make it difficult or impossible for us to achieve a sense of well-being.
2. The feelings, in their emotional dimension—which make us experience what our internal and external worlds offer us. Faced with a threat to the integrality of being, this dimension can be a way of reorganizing us in the face of this possibility of death, but it can also be the main agent of our greatest suffering.
3. Intimate relationships, in their family dimension—which characterizes us as gregarious beings, making us feel part of an important group.
4. Supporting relationships, in their social dimension.
5. The essence of the human being, in its spiritual dimension.

We believe it is the physician's duty to understand that suffering is more feared than death and that it is a priority to provide comfort and relief from pain and other symptoms that cause identifiable suffering (Fig. 6.1).

A systematic review of studies focused on cancer, acquired immunodeficiency syndrome (AIDS), heart disease, chronic obstructive pulmonary disease (COPD),

A. C. L. Q. Arantes, *Clinical Assessment of Human Suffering*,
https://doi.org/10.1007/978-3-030-57535-9_6

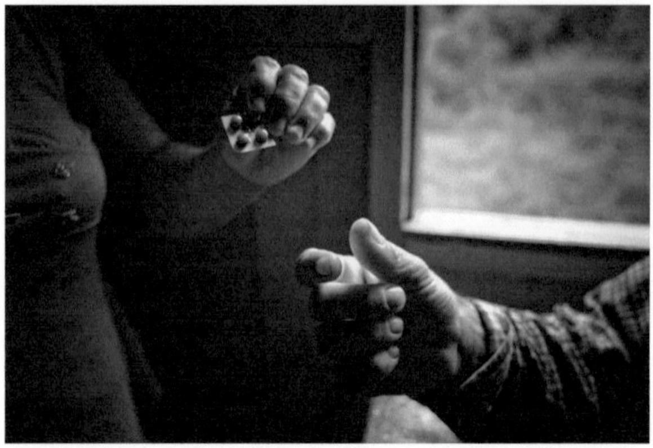

Fig. 6.1 The physician should provide comfort and relief from pain and other symptoms that cause identifiable suffering

and chronic kidney disease identified eleven of the most prevalent symptoms in terminally ill patients: pain, depression, anxiety, confusion, fatigue, shortness of breath, insomnia, nausea, constipation, diarrhea, and anorexia [1].

The clinician must understand the patient's priorities and goals for symptom relief. A convenient way to ascertain individual expectations is to ask the patient to rate their degree of suffering on a scale [2] and determine the level of relief desired; this can be expressed numerically, descriptively, or as an acceptable level of interference with daily functioning activities. Regardless of the intensity of the symptom classification, asking about and better assessing the patient's "most problematic" symptom reveals additional and potentially more disturbing burdens in almost a third of patients in palliative care [3, 4].

Patients at an advanced stage of a serious illness that threatens the continuity of life usually have several symptoms, the most common of which are pain, depression, anxiety, confusion, fatigue, shortness of breath, insomnia, nausea, constipation, diarrhea, and anorexia [5, 6].

The importance of symptom assessment is becoming increasingly apparent. In a seminal study, cancer patients undergoing treatment had better health-related quality of life [7] and longer survival (31 months versus 26 months) [8] when given the ability to self-assess and report their symptoms (as "patient-reported results") to the oncology team.

Patients who have many symptoms are said to have a high symptom load. These symptoms can result from several factors. Among patients with advanced cancer, for example, symptoms may result from the disease (for example, bone pain due to metastases or dyspnea due to pleural effusion), treatment (for example, esophagitis with chest radiotherapy), or other concomitant conditions (for example, osteoarthritis).

Each identified symptom should be investigated for its intensity, onset, duration, alleviating factors, exacerbating factors, and other related symptoms. It is also important to understand the personal meaning of a symptom for the patient and how it affects their psychosocial well-being. The following are sample questions that can be used to explore the meaning of specific symptoms:

- "Of the symptoms that bother you, which symptom bothers you the most?" This will identify a primary symptom in one third of patients, which would otherwise go unrecognized [3].
- "How does this symptom affect you? How much does it interfere with your life—for example, your sleep, your daily activities, and your sense of well-being?"
- "What thoughts do you have about the meaning of this symptom?"
- "Does this symptom make you worry about your health and your illness? What are your concerns?"
- "How does this symptom affect your family and friends?"

Discussing symptoms with the patient's caregivers can also be informative and can offer opportunities for support and education for the patient's family and friends [9].

After the initial assessment, periodic reassessment of symptoms is valuable for identifying or modifying treatment goals, monitoring the response to specific symptomatic interventions, and communicating between members of the health team and with caregivers.

The dimensions of symptom assessment are different aspects of symptoms, such as their severity, their frequency, their level of interference in activities, and the level of suffering associated with these symptoms.

The severity of symptoms is a useful guide to treatment (for example, a need for pain relief) and can also provide prognostic information (for example, the presence of dyspnea).

The use of classification instruments completed by the patients themselves represents a major change in the assessment of symptoms in the last 30 years. When assessing symptoms, it is useful to ascertain the patient's severity rating over a given period, such as the last 24 hours. This approach to classifying pain depends solely on how the patient reports the pain, using a verbal or numerical scale. The patient may be asked to stretch a stretcher along a 10 cm straight line (a visual analogue scale (VAS)) or rate the severity on a scale from 0 to 10, where 10 is the worst. These approaches are based on psychophysical studies in the field of subjective sensory physiology, which demonstrated that the perception of a stimulus is closely related to the strength of the stimulus [10]. For many symptoms, however, there is no clear evidence of the ideal cutoff points to define the severity of symptoms [11].

Some patients are unable to assess the severity of their symptoms on a numerical scale [12]. An alternative approach is to ask patients to rate the distress caused by their symptoms, instead of their severity, and give them categories of response (for example, "They don't bother me a bit" or "They bother me a little" or "They bother me a lot"). Some symptoms, such as fatigue, can be classified by patients as mild in severity but severe in terms of suffering. The amount and type of interference with daily activities caused by a symptom can also illustrate the severity of the symptoms and provide another means of determining therapeutic success.

We consider that we have many challenges in assessment of and care for physical suffering:

- The patient's assessment of symptoms may differ from that of the health care professional. In general, doctors (and caregivers) have greater disagreement with patients in assessing the severity of subjective symptoms than that of objective states, such as the presence of vomiting. The severity of symptoms tends to be classified as less severe by doctors than by patients and family members, and doctors tend to expect patients to tolerate levels of suffering and symptoms that patients consider unacceptable [13–15]. On the other hand, family members also tend to exaggerate symptoms [16, 17]. However, with regard to pain, older family members tend to exaggerate it, while younger ones tend to underestimate it [16].
- Patients may underestimate or not report symptoms (mainly pain) because they fear that worsening of symptoms will reflect the progression of their disease and that the oncologist will interrupt their treatment. Underreporting can also occur if a patient feels that a symptom, such as pain, is an inevitable consequence of the disease, its treatment, or dying. In addition, if patients do not receive attention to their most frequent complaints, they can stop communicating about problems related to those specific complaints.
- Symptoms may change over time.
- Many symptoms are of multifactorial origin.
- Patients and/or their families may have had adverse experiences in the health system and lost confidence in the system and/or caregivers. This can make them particularly reluctant to discuss psychological symptoms. Particularly in these cases, the evaluation interview with the patient and the family can, in itself, have therapeutic value in improving the caregiver's relationship with the patient and the family, eliciting care preferences and developing trust.
- Cultural factors can determine which symptoms are acceptable for discussion between patients and doctors, and how patients perceive their symptoms. For example, women from particular cultures may not be comfortable discussing gynecological complaints with a male doctor [18].

6.1.1 Evaluation and Classification Instruments for Symptoms

Formal multiple symptom assessment tools, especially those that are symptom inventories (such as the Edmonton Symptom Assessment System—Revised (ESAS-r) [19]), provide a good overview of symptoms in individual patients.

In particular, several symptom assessment tools are highly effective in recognizing unreported symptoms when combined with new patient interviews to obtain further details about positive responses. When a specific tool is chosen, it must be used consistently to ensure reliability in the clinical environment.

Many of these symptom assessment tools have been tested for reliability and validity. However, as with any other measure of health outcomes, errors can occur in the assessment [20]. The possibilities for evaluation errors include the following:

- Motor, hearing, and visual impairments may impede the utility of symptom assessment tools in older adults [21].
- Cognitive dysfunction can lead to misleading responses and inaccurate assessment, even when the assessment is combined with behavioral indicators [22]. Cognitive dysfunction can be quite subtle.
- Shorter assessment tools can overlook symptoms that are important to the patient, and longer assessment tools can be too tiring for patients to complete.
- As the patient's condition changes, the classification of symptoms may change as they adapt to the new condition, even if specific symptoms have not changed. This is called the *response change phenomenon*. Classifications can also be influenced by other symptoms, especially anxiety and other emotional reactions, which may change over time.
- The interpretation of the anchors at both ends of the scale (for example, 0 and 10 on a numerical scale from 0 to 10) may vary between patients, depending on their previous experience. Caregivers and health professionals can also interpret anchors differently. It may be necessary to repeat the anchor definitions when asking patients to give a rating.
- In numerical scales, the cutoff point is a number that identifies how to categorize severity. Studies have identified cutoff points of 4 out of 10 (mild versus moderate) and 7 out of 10 (moderate versus severe) for pain [23]. For other symptoms, these cutoff point values are still being studied.

Despite these limitations, several validated multiple symptom assessment tools are widely used in palliative and end-of-life care settings, including:

- The Edmonton Symptom Assessment System—Revised (ESAS-r) [19]
- The Memorial Symptom Assessment Scale—Short Form (MSAS-SF) and the Condensed Memorial Symptom Assessment Scale (CMSAS) [24, 25]
- The MD Anderson Symptom Inventory (MDASI) [26, 27]
- The Rotterdam Symptom Checklist (RSCL) [27]
- The Symptom Distress Scale (SDS) [28]

6.2 The Emotional Dimension

The main psychological symptoms that require evaluation in patients in palliative care are depression (as distinct from the adjustment and grief reaction), anxiety, and delirium. Physicians should assess multiple factors that increase the prevalence and/or the severity of psychological distress (for example, rapidly advancing illness, use of medications such as interferon or glucocorticoids, metabolic abnormalities, uncontrolled pain, impaired cognition, and financial problems) and address them, if possible. Psychological suffering often decreases with adequate pain relief [29].

Sadness, depression, and demoralization There is a high frequency of mood disorders in patients with a serious and/or life-threatening illness. As an example, in one meta-analysis performed in patients receiving palliative care, the combined prevalence of all types of depression was 25% and the prevalence of mood disorders was 38% [30]. The spectrum of mood disorders and conditions seen in patients in palliative care includes sadness, a normal reaction to grief (including anticipatory grief), pathological grief, adjustment disorder with depressed characteristics, minor and major depression, and demoralization.

Grief versus depression Grief—a natural and expected reaction to a life-limiting disease and loss—can and should be differentiated from major depression [31].

Unfortunately, depression is often unrecognized and undiagnosed in patients receiving palliative care [14, 32]. The prevalence, burden, and challenges in recognizing and treating depression in palliative care patients are addressed in detail elsewhere.

Patients with advanced disease can exhibit many of the vegetative signs of depression (sleep disorders, poor concentration, fatigue, poor appetite) without becoming depressed, as these symptoms can be caused by the medical condition or treatment. Patients facing the end of life can also demonstrate significant guilt and concern about death without becoming depressed. However, the presence of these markers in the absence of other causes should lead to suspicion of depression. Indicators of poor emotional well-being—such as a sense of general hopelessness, helplessness, worthlessness, or guilt—can be more useful for diagnosing and assessing suicide risk. Unrelieved symptoms, especially pain, can contribute to a feeling of hopelessness and lead to depression among patients with severe pain or other symptoms (Fig. 6.2).

The impact of mood disorders on palliative care is highlighted by a study that found that mortality rates in cancer patients are up to 25% higher in those who have depressive symptoms [33]. In addition, individuals who suffer from depression are at increased risk of suicide. Passive suicidal ideation ("I would be better off dead") must be distinguished from active suicidal ideation ("I would be better off dead, and this is how I'm going to do it"). An expressed wish for a hasty death should be

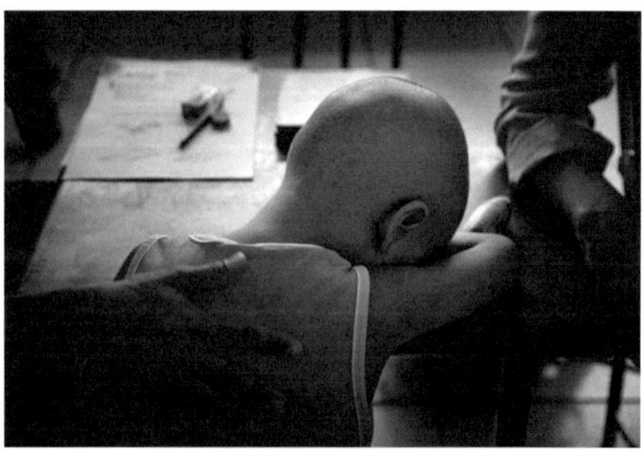

Fig. 6.2 Patients with advanced disease can exhibit signs of depression

considered not a request for euthanasia but a marker of intense anguish that requires further exploration [34].

Screening using a simple assessment via a question ("Are you depressed?" or "Have you been depressed most of the time in the last 2 weeks?") has a negative predictive value (NPV) of 94% [35, 36] in identification of patients in whom a diagnosis of depression would be excluded on the basis of a complete psychiatric interview. Addition of a second question that addresses anhedonia ("Have you experienced a loss of interest in things or activities that you would normally enjoy?") increases the NPV to 98% [36].

It is important to note that these brief tools are designed for screening patients and identifying those who subsequently need a complete diagnostic evaluation for depression.

Demoralization Demoralization is a state of mind with reduced morale and deficient coping, characterized by feelings of hopelessness, helplessness, and loss of purpose and meaning; it is distinct from clinical depression [37] and may be precipitated by existential suffering [38]. On the other hand, depression is a loss of pleasure and interest in the present moment (generalized anhedonia).

Demoralization is a common problem among patients with serious medical conditions. A systematic review found that the prevalence of demoralization is about 15% in patients with cancer and progressive disease [39]. Despite this, there is a general lack of awareness of demoralization and how and when to intervene [159]. Among the factors that are consistently associated with demoralization are poorly controlled physical symptoms, inadequately treated depression and anxiety, reduced social functioning, unemployment, marital status [37], and possibly age and sex [40].

Treatment of demoralization in patients receiving palliative care may include restoring some control (for example, through better pain control) or providing meaning (for example, through cognitive–behavioral therapy, life review, dignity therapy, and meaning-centered psychotherapy). More research is needed in this area [38].

Anxiety Anxiety is common in patients with severe or life-threatening advanced disease. As an example, the reported prevalence of anxiety among patients with advanced cancer is 18% [41].

Anxiety can also be related to a pre-existing anxiety disorder, substance abuse, delirium, or undertreated symptoms—most commonly, pain. A single aggregate question ("Have you been anxious, nervous, uncomfortable, tense, or scared in the past few days?") can be used to track symptoms of anxiety.

Delirium Delirium and confusional states are among the most common neuropsychiatric disorders found in patients with medical conditions, particularly older individuals. According to the 2013 edition of the American Psychiatric Association's *Diagnostic and Statistical Manual of Mental Disorders* (DSM-5), the diagnosis of delirium requires all of the following criteria to be met [42]:

- Attention and awareness disorders that develop quickly (usually within hours to days) and tend to fluctuate each day
- Cognition disorders (for example, in memory, orientation, language, visual spatial capacity, and/or perception)

- Disorders in attention, awareness, and cognition that are not better explained by another neurocognitive disorder and do not occur in the context of a coma
- Evidence from the patient's history, physical examination, or laboratory findings indicating that the disorders are caused by a general medical condition, intoxication, withdrawal from substances, and/or side effects of medication

The subtypes of delirium are delineated on the basis of the patient's psychomotor behavior and level of arousal [42, 43].

- Hypoactive subtype: Psychomotor retardation, lethargy, and a decreased level of arousal.
- Hyperactive subtype: Restlessness, agitation, and hypervigilance. Humor, lack of cooperation with care, and psychotic characteristics may also be present.

The mnemonic FACT provides a summary of the diagnostic criteria for delirium:

- *F*luctuating cognitive deficit(s) with acute onset
- *A*ttention deficit
- *C*onsciousness level disturbance
- *T*houghts that are disorganized

Delirium is the most common neuropsychiatric complication seen in patients with advanced cancer near the end of life and can result in suffering for patients, families, and health professionals. It is also a marker of reduced survival in hospitalized and institutionalized patients [44–46].

Delirium in cancer patients is often overlooked and often diagnosed as akathisia, anxiety, dementia, depression, or psychosis [47, 48].

For many terminal patients with COPD, end-stage renal disease, heart failure, or other serious life-threatening illnesses, global brain dysfunction without a definable reversible cause, manifested as delirium, is the common final complication that precedes death. However, for many patients in palliative care, several factors can contribute to development of delirium, many of which are potentially reversible [49].

Many of the risk factors for delirium are already present in patients with advanced terminal illnesses, although many patients improve with treatment of specific causes. The fact that delirium is reversible in up to 50% of cases [49] highlights the importance of early recognition and aggressive assessment and management.

The Bedside Confusion Scale (which tests the patient's ability to recite the 12 months in reverse order and assesses their state of consciousness) is another excellent tool for tracking and longitudinally following delirium in palliative care [50]. Adding sevens in series and spelling a word such as "farm" or "world" backward are other simple tests of attention.

6.3 The Family Dimension

One of the goals of palliative care is to provide psychosocial support for patients and families in the face of potentially fatal diseases. Psychosocial care can be defined as "concern for the psychological aspects and emotional well-being of the

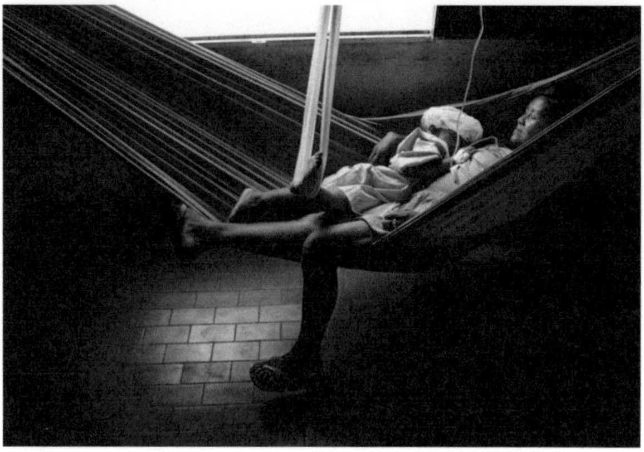

Fig. 6.3 The culture of the patient is also considered during care

patient and [their] family caregivers, including issues related to [their] self-esteem, adequate communication, and knowledge and acceptance of the disease" [51].

In palliative care, it is considered that the patient, their family, and their loved ones are the focus of attention. The well-being of the family's present and future is strongly affected by the care provided for the patient. Caregivers can be a mix of family, friends, volunteers, and health professionals. They are people who are intimately involved with the patient and who love them. These people can be defined by the patient as those who can advise on decision making and emotional support [52] (Fig. 6.3).

In general, a family can be understood as two or more people who usually live in the same abode, have an emotional or affective bond, and perform interrelated social tasks [53]—or even as a relationship in which people live together, are committed, form an economic unit, care for the youngest of them, and identify with each other and with the group to which they belong [53]. Nowadays, one of the most accepted definitions of a patient's family is that it includes those whom the patient defines as their family, or it is even said that "Binominal is who its members say they are" [54].

In the context of palliative care, we can also use the *mobile model* to better understand the dynamics of the patient–family binomial: "The family is like a mobile and each member is represented by a toy piece. The sum of the pieces forms the whole and, in turn, all of them, however different they may be, are made to occupy a place whose common result is balance. Illness and death work as events that unbalance the family system, as if someone removed a piece from the mobile. In this way, everything that affects each individual will also affect the family as a whole" (Fig. 6.4).

From the moment when the diagnosis is received, there is a change in the family balance, which intensifies even more with the proximity of the patient's death [54, 55].

The current trend in many countries is to suggest that patients stay in their homes, under the care of their family. The delicate relationship between the caregiver and the individual at the end of life allows us to infer that humanization often does not occur. "It is not necessarily the place that humanizes the therapeutic relationship but

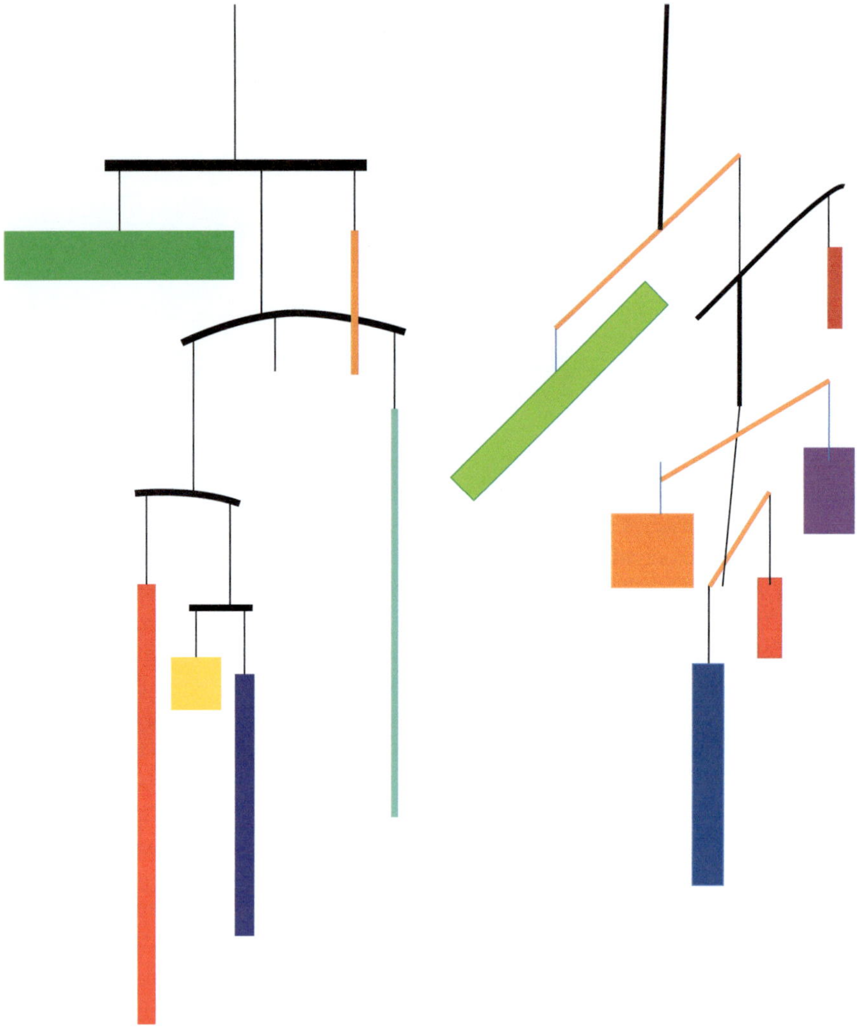

Fig. 6.4 Each member of a family is represented by a toy piece in a mobile. Illness and death may unbalance the family system, as if someone removed a piece from the mobile

the empathic interest that the professional develops for the patient" [56]. If the objective is to improve the quality of care offered, it is essential to recognize the needs of the family and of formal and informal caregivers, and to establish support strategies for them.

Families who care for patients near the end of life may experience often challenging and sometimes conflicting experiences. Caregiving responsibilities can include medical and physical tasks, managing finances, patient advocacy, decision making, emotional support, and coordination of care. Studies show that caring can have negative consequences for these families, including fatigue, problems related to sleep, depression, anxiety, weight loss, burnout, and increased risk of mortality.

These families face not only demands related to care but also the sadness and loss associated with the impending death of their relative [53]. Study of the burden associated with the caregiver—be it of a "physical" or "mental" cause—is a priority in palliative care, since it allows assessment of the negative consequences for the caregiver and, consequently, the possible repercussions for the patient [57, 58].

In fact, family members may need as much or more support than the patient themselves, as they are facing an imminent loss, experiencing anticipatory mourning, trying to offer emotional support to the patient, feeling guilty, concerned about the aftermath, and still overwhelmed with the patient's care.

Self care Although the quality of life of family members is often the same as that of the patient, other elements are also relevant [58]. Some studies show that the quality of life of family members is affected by the patient's needs: "I must give the patient the best care I can, and they are doing their best for me." Thus, the key to the quality-of-life aspects of family members is that the patient is comfortable [53].

Families and informal caregivers need information and guidance about the individual's illness and how to care for it, in addition to psychological and social support. Being well informed about the disease seems to decrease anxiety and possible fears, which are sometimes unlikely or unfounded. As the vast majority of family members and informal caregivers do not have training in nursing, they benefit from practical instructions on how to administer medications and how to change the patient's position in bed, among other things [56].

Certain studies have reported favorable results of interventions with specific targets, such as insomnia therapies and problem-solving skills training, as well as definition of clear goals and interventions, assessment of the specific needs of the caregiver, preventive interventions, and facilitation of the positive aspects of caregiving [52].

In a systematic review on the existing instruments related to the family caregiver in palliative care, Hudson et al. showed that there is a lack of coherence in the way the needs of family caregivers are generally assessed, since there have been too few longitudinal studies that have analyzed the impacts of providing care and too few evidence-based interventions that have assessed and actually responded to the needs of family members [51].

To make a family assessment, it is important to ask:

- "What are the needs of this family?"
- "What resources do they have, and what resources do they need to find?"

6.4 The Social Dimension

Proper assessment of the social dimension must answer the following question: "Is there a social problem and, if so, why has it not been resolved?" Therefore, it is necessary to assess what is needed that will meet the demands of the patient and their family. Eventually, a solution to social problems can be achieved through one or more interventions, such as providing information, improving internal family

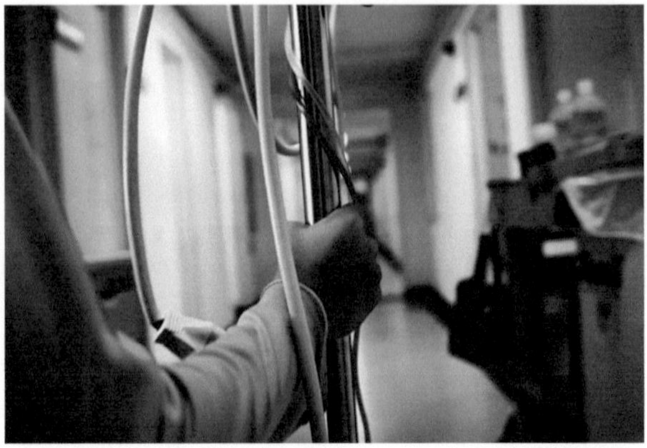

Fig. 6.5 It is essential to provide not only information but also alternative resources for patients and their families

communication, encouraging and supporting initiatives, or offering material resources [59] (Fig. 6.5).

Almost a third of the families of critically ill adults report loss of all or most of their savings as a result of the illness and the need for care [60]. In addition, the financial burden can have a profound impact on health care decisions.

In one study, the family's financial difficulties were associated with a preference for comfortable care over long-term care [61]; in another, substantial care needs were associated with a greater likelihood of terminally ill patients considering euthanasia or physician-assisted death [62].

With regard to the social perspective, we first seek to meet with the patient, their family, and their caregivers. It is necessary to draw a socioeconomic profile with information that will be fundamental in the management of the case. Thus, it is important to recognize the family with whom we will keep in touch exactly as it is (real family) and not as we would like it to be (the ideal family) [63]. Family bonds have not always been formed satisfactorily; it is not always the case that the dying person is "loved by everyone"; the family does not always have adequate financial, emotional, and/or organizational conditions to care for the patient; and the patient does not always want to be cared for in the way we consider ideal or necessary.

Knowing and understanding the family and its limits and possibilities is the first step toward adequate care; for this, listening and welcoming are essential actions, as well as recognizing the appropriate moment for the approach. We will not hear everything in the first interview and we will not notice much in the first approach. For this reason, it is essential that the social service professional knows the right way and the right time to gather information, and knows the appropriate time to just listen and be welcoming.

With regard to socioeconomic assessment, some information is essential and must be obtained in the first approach—for example, the composition of the patient's family and their place of residence, income, spiritual beliefs, training, profession, and employment situation. These data will support social assistance, as they provide adequate parameters regarding the needs experienced by the family and/or show their mechanisms for coping with limitations. Schematically, we can describe the family's composition; with whom the patient resides and whom they can (or cannot) count on for care; whether the family is extended or nuclear; whether it is a single-parent family [64]; and whether there are other individuals in the same family nucleus who require specific care (such as children, dependent elderly people, or other sick individuals). These data will help us to assist the family in the search for alternatives when the available care is not sufficient for the patient's needs.

Place of residence This is also related to the need to understand the social support network. Depending on where the individual resides, it is necessary to understand whether their social support network is precarious or sufficient, as well as whether it is easy or difficult for them to attend appointments for consultations or procedures. Awareness of these difficulties or facilities enables the social worker to facilitate matters by arranging appropriate referrals to resources in the region, arranging transportation from other institutions, or seeking home assistance through the institution itself or through the neighborhood/municipality where the patient resides, depending on the degree of difficulties encountered by the family in attending scheduled appointments or providing the required home care.

Training, professional, and employment situation of the patient This information is essential, especially when the family is reliant on the patient's income. Orientation and appropriate referral to the relevant resources will provide a guarantee of support for the family unit.

Family income This is closely related to the previous item and is not always accorded sufficient importance in the analysis. It is always important for this information to be known so the team has real parameters for future requests. Requirements beyond what the family can afford—in this instance, specifically related to costs—tend to make patient care unfeasible and generate unnecessarily stressful situations for those involved.

Spiritual beliefs This is a very important cultural aspect in social assessment of a patient in palliative care. The spiritual beliefs of the family and the patient inform appropriate approaches to the patient's death, care at the end of life, rituals, and different needs related to personal beliefs and meanings. This should be known and shared with the team so that, as far as possible, the patient's care at the end of life is adjusted to what is significant and symbolic for the family and the patient.

Social support network This relates to entities (institutions, formal groups, and services) or people (relatives, friends, and neighbors) on whom the patient and his family can count in the event of need. The sufficiency and effectiveness of support networks depend on how much availability and security they offer to individuals who use them; such effectiveness is related not to the income of those involved but, rather, to the bonds established and strengthened over time [65].

Institution Here we refer specifically to the institution to which the palliative care service is linked. It is part of the work objectives of the social worker to get to know, in depth, the institution in which they carry out their work. This knowledge will provide conditions for the professional to find out about the available services and the client's referral channels. The social worker needs to know how to create their own intrainstitutional network in order to serve patients well, and to know if a single service is not able to meet all of the requirements of those who need care, even if it is part of a large institution. Knowing the interfaces, establishing partnerships, knowing the proper referral channels, and fast-tracking the engagement of the appropriate services with the patient are also parts of the social worker's role in the palliative care group.

It is part of the multidimensional evaluation to evaluate the social support network of those involved so they can be enabled to activate it in appropriate situations; to know and establish a support network within the institution in which the patient is being attended, in order to ensure accurate patient care; and to be an interlocutor between the patient/family and staff regarding issues related to cultural and social aspects that involve care in general. Added to this is the importance of listening and being welcoming at such a special time—the time of coping with an incurable disease and the final stage of life.

6.5 The Spiritual Dimension

Spirituality may well have an ontology [66, 67]. However, whatever ontology it may seem to have, it is clear that it has been interpreted in various ways and that the context in which these interpretive actions take place is significant. The point is that understandings of spirituality are inevitably influenced—and, to some extent, constructed—by the social context within which they are developed. Spirituality is constructed in different ways by various religious traditions, spiritual movements, belief systems, cultures, contexts, and—not least—individuals in specific circumstances. Everyone can use the term "spirituality" but different people can use it in very different ways. Our point is that spirituality is not only a social or cultural means to be considered. Likewise, the question of whether our understandings of spirituality have natural or supernatural roots [68] is not the issue here. The point is that spirituality is never given to us as a kind of tightly wrapped gift, which we unpack and can apply to all places at all times and in all circumstances. On the contrary, the meaning of spirituality is necessarily emergent and dialectical; it is shaped and formed by the context within which spiritual language is expressed. At this point, we can relate to a virtue that is especially necessary for health professionals: cultural humility. Culturally appropriate care allows physicians to provide respectful services and respond to the linguistic health beliefs, practices, and needs of diverse patients. This care ideally demonstrates "cultural humility" [69], which goes beyond the discrete domain of a body of fixed and finite knowledge [70]. Cultural humility is defined as a process of openness and self-awareness, into which self-reflection and criticism are incorporated after interaction with different individuals [71] Cultural humility recognizes that culture is changeable over time and defined in a unique way in the context of a patient's life experiences and beliefs. It requires the clinician's active involvement and curiosity about each patient as a person, including how the patient fits into their broader cultural community. It also requires physicians to reflect on how their own culture and the culture of contemporary biomedicine [72] may interact with the patient's culture to influence patient care and the doctor–patient relationship [69, 73, 74]. As an example, medical values about the importance of detachment and the objectivity of the doctor can represent barriers to culturally appropriate care, especially for minorities. Several barriers to high-quality care at the end of life of minority patients have been identified, one of which is failure on the part of health professionals to provide culturally appropriate care that considers differences in cultural attitudes toward suffering and death, various decision-making styles, varied family roles, and patient and family preferences regarding information sharing [75, 76].

An impending health crisis causes a patient to examine their personal values, their relationships, and the meanings of life and death. Life-threatening illness evokes questions such as "Why me?" and "Is there anything that transcends death?" Therefore, in addition to assessing spirituality and religious beliefs, the tasks involved in palliative care assessment include assessment of hopes and fears, meaning, purpose, beliefs about life after death, guilt, forgiveness, and life review and completion. Open-ended questions should be asked, such as "Probing questions" and "What do I need to know about you as a person to provide the best care possible?" This approach can facilitate the initial assessment in this field [77].

Many patients hold denominational beliefs that can have a profound impact on their medical care, including beliefs about transfusions, mechanical ventilation, hydration and nutrition, the role of miracles, and physician-assisted death. For example, a high level of confidence in religious faith to deal with cancer has been associated with greater use of intensive care near the time of death [78]. Since most oncologists do not consider it their role to provide spiritual assistance [79], it is imperative that a structured palliative care assessment investigates spiritual/existential beliefs and guides shared decision making between the doctor and the patient (Fig. 6.6).

Along with the prescriptive impact of spiritual principles, the importance of spirituality in coping with disease is endorsed by most cancer patients; for example, in one study, patients who prayed or meditated and those visited by a spiritual adviser reported a higher quality of life [80]. Many, however, report insufficient levels of spiritual support from their communities and the medical system [81] in the last

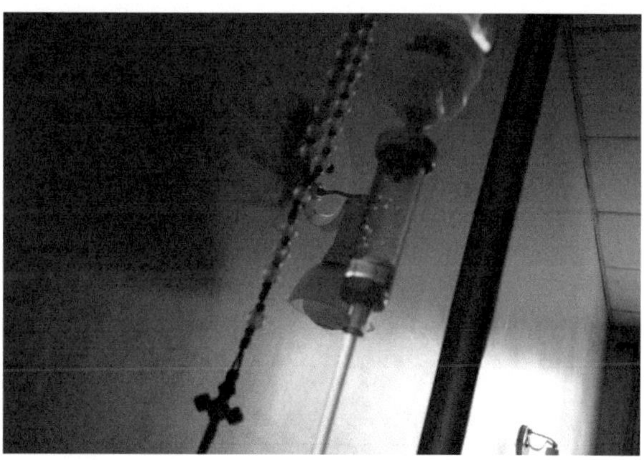

Fig. 6.6 A patient's beliefs can have a profound impact on their medical care

weeks of life—a characteristic associated with an increased likelihood of receiving aggressive and nonbeneficial treatment measures at the end of life [82].

To assess the relevance of spirituality or religion and the patient's needs in this dimension [81, 83], the initial screening process may use questions such as:

- "Are spirituality or religion important in your life?"
- "Are your spiritual/religious needs being met?"
- "Are you at peace?"

The final step—spiritual evaluation—is best performed by a trained spiritual adviser or counselor and should be carried out with open dialogue and empathic listening. It may include exploratory and interpretative questions such as:

- "Where do you find the strength to face your illness?"
- "Are you scared of the idea of dying?"
- "Have you ever wondered if God has abandoned you?"
- "Has your faith/religion ever caused you stress or conflict?"

Physicians should be particularly sensitive to comments that may indicate spiritual distress. Often, patients express spiritual need through comments that suggest fear, despair, guilt, a desire for a hasty death, or hopelessness. For example, a previous history of conflict or stress related to faith/religion is associated with increased symptoms of anxiety and depression in patients with advanced disease [84], and this can lead to refusal of potentially effective therapies, on the one hand, or to insistence on nonbeneficial interventions, on the other.

Assessing the transcendent needs of nonreligious or nonspiritual patients requires sensitivity that can go beyond a methodology or protocol. The concerns of atheist patients are often of a moral and/or humanistic nature and can be assessed, as long as the provider maintains respect for rationalism and disbelief, and refrains from making references to God. The assessment can be facilitated by use of interview questions that communicate compassion and concern, such as:

- "This type of illness often raises important questions. . . . How are you dealing with it?"

Another aspect of the transcendent domain assessment concerns a life review. Common themes include completion of the patient's life matters, contributions to others, and legacy; concerns about these tasks arise with diagnosis of a disease that limits life [85]. Evaluation and facilitation of the life review can be implemented as a sequence of evaluation questions and facilitated responses from the patient, in a process similar to dignity therapy [84]:

- "How would you like to be remembered?"
- "What are you most proud of (in your life)?"
- "Do you feel prepared for what is still ahead of you?"
- "What do you still want to accomplish in your life?"
- "Have you been able to share lessons, thoughts, and important things with others?"
- "Are there any specific things you feel you still need to say to your loved ones?"

Doctors should recognize, however, that patients may not want to talk to their doctors about these matters.

References

1. Moens K, Higginson IJ, Harding R, EURO IMPACT. Are there differences in the prevalence of palliative care-related problems in people living with advanced cancer and eight non-cancer conditions? A systematic review. J Pain Symptom Manage. 2014;48(4):660–77. https://doi.org/10.1016/j.jpainsymman.2013.11.009.
2. Strömgren AS, Sjogren P, Goldschmidt D, Petersen MA, Pedersen L, Groenvold M. Symptom priority and course of symptomatology in specialized palliative care. J Pain Symptom Manage. 2006;31(3):199–206. https://doi.org/10.1016/j.jpainsymman.2005.07.007.
3. Hoekstra J, Vernooij-Dassen MJ, de Vos R, Bindels PJ. The added value of assessing the 'most troublesome' symptom among patients with cancer in the palliative phase. Patient Educ Couns. 2007;65(2):223–9. https://doi.org/10.1016/j.pec.2006.08.001.
4. Li B, Mah K, Swami N, Pope A, Hannon B, Lo C, Rodin G, Le LW, Zimmermann C. Symptom assessment in patients with advanced cancer: are the most severe symptoms the most bothersome? J Palliat Med. 2019;22(10):1252–9. https://doi.org/10.1089/jpm.2018.0622.
5. Reuben DB, Mor V, Hiris J. Clinical symptoms and length of survival in patients with terminal cancer. Arch Intern Med. 1988;148(7):1586–91.
6. Walsh D, Donnelly S, Rybicki L. The symptoms of advanced cancer: relationship to age, gender, and performance status in 1,000 patients. Support Care Cancer. 2000;8(3):175–9. https://doi.org/10.1007/s005200050281.
7. Basch E, Deal AM, Kris MG, Scher HI, Hudis CA, Sabbatini P, Rogak L, Bennett AV, Dueck AC, Atkinson TM, Chou JF, Dulko D, Sit L, Barz A, Novotny P, Fruscione M, Sloan JA, Schrag D. Symptom monitoring with patient-reported outcomes during routine cancer treatment: a randomized controlled trial. J Clin Oncol. 2016;34(6):557–65. https://doi.org/10.1200/JCO.2015.63.0830. Errata in: J Clin Oncol. 2016; 34 (18): 2198 and J Clin Oncol. 2019; 37 (6): 528.
8. Basch E, Deal AM, Dueck AC, Scher HI, Kris MG, Hudis C, Schrag D. Overall survival results of a trial assessing patient-reported outcomes for symptom monitoring during routine cancer treatment. JAMA. 2017;318(2):197–8. https://doi.org/10.1001/jama.2017.7156.
9. Mehta A, Ezer H. My love hurts: the meaning that spouses attribute to the pain of their loved ones during palliative care. J Palliat Care. 2003;19(2):87–94. https://doi.org/10.1177/082585970301900203.
10. Dudel J. General sensory physiology, psychophysics. In: Schmidt RF, editor. Fundamentals of sensory physiology. 1st ed. Berlin: Springer; 1978. p. 1–30.
11. Oldenmenger WH, de Raaf PJ, de Klerk C, van der Rijt CC. Cut points on 0–10 numeric rating scales for symptoms included in the Edmonton Symptom Assessment Scale in cancer patients: a systematic review. J Pain Symptom Manage. 2013;45(6):1083–93. https://doi.org/10.1016/j.jpainsymman.2012.06.007.
12. Sze FK, Chung TK, Wong E, Lam KK, Lo R, Woo J. Pain in Chinese cancer patients under palliative care. Palliat Med. 1998;12(4):271–7. https://doi.org/10.1191/026921698666535718.
13. Grossman SA, Sheidler VR, Swedeen K, Mucenski J, Piantadosi S. Correlation of patient and caregiver ratings of cancer pain. J Pain Symptom Manage. 1991;6(2):53–7. https://doi.org/10.1016/0885-3924(91)90518-9.
14. Passik SD, Dugan W, McDonald MV, Rosenfeld B, Theobald DE, Edgerton S. Oncologists' recognition of depression in their patients with cancer. J Clin Oncol. 1998;16(4):1594–600. https://doi.org/10.1200/JCO.1998.16.4.1594.
15. Marquié L, Raufaste E, Lauque D, Mariné C, Ecoiffier M, Sorum P. Pain rating by patients and physicians: evidence of systematic pain miscalibration. Pain. 2003;102(3):289–96. https://doi.org/10.1016/s0304-3959(02)00402-5.

16. Kurtz ME, Kurtz JC, Given CC, Given B. Concordance of cancer patient and caregiver symptom reports. Cancer Pract. 1996;4(4):185–90.
17. Silveira MJ, Given CW, Given B, Rosland AM, Piette JD. Patient–caregiver concordance in symptom assessment and improvement in outcomes for patients undergoing cancer chemotherapy. Chronic Illn. 2010;6(1):46–56. https://doi.org/10.1177/1742395309359208.
18. Koffman J, Morgan M, Edmonds P, Speck P, Higginson I. Cultural meanings of pain: a qualitative study of Black Caribbean and White British patients with advanced cancer. Palliat Med. 2008;22(4):350–9. https://doi.org/10.1177/0269216308090168.
19. Watanabe SM, Nekolaichuk C, Beaumont C, Johnson L, Myers J, Strasser F. A multicenter study comparing two numerical versions of the Edmonton Symptom Assessment System in palliative care patients. J Pain Symptom Manage. 2011;41(2):456–68. https://doi.org/10.1016/j.jpainsymman.2010.04.020.
20. Hahn EA, Cella D, Chassany O, Fairclough DL, Wong GY. Hays RD; Clinical Significance Consensus Meeting Group. Precision of health-related quality-of-life data compared with other clinical measures. Mayo Clin Proc. 2007;82(10):1244–54. https://doi.org/10.4065/82.10.1244.
21. Jacox A, Carr DB, Payne R, Berde CB, Breitbart W, Cain JM, Chapman CR, Cleeland CS, Ferrell BR, Finley RS, Hester NO, Hill CS, Leak WD, Lipman AG, Logan CL, McGarvey CL, Miaskowski CA, Mulder DS, Paice JA, Shapiro BS, Silberstein EB, Smith RS, Stover J, Tsou CV, Vecchiarelli L, Weissman DE. Management of cancer pain: clinical practice guideline no. 9. AHCPR publication no. 94-0592. Agency for Health Care Policy and Research: Rockville; 1994.
22. Coyle N, Breitbart W, Weaver S, Portenoy R. Delirium as a contributing factor to "crescendo" pain: three case reports. J Pain Symptom Manage. 1994;9(1):44–7. https://doi.org/10.1016/0885-3924(94)90146-5.
23. Serlin RC, Mendoza TR, Nakamura Y, Edwards KR, Cleeland CS. When is cancer pain mild, moderate or severe? Grading pain severity by its interference with function. Pain. 1995;61(2):277–84. https://doi.org/10.1016/0304-3959(94)00178-h.
24. Chang VT, Hwang SS, Feuerman M, Kasimis BS, Thaler HT. The Memorial Symptom Assessment Scale Short Form (MSAS-SF). Cancer. 2000;89(5):1162–71. https://doi.org/10.1002/1097-0142(20000901)89:5<1162::aid-cncr26>3.0.co;2-y.
25. Chang VT, Hwang SS, Kasimis B, Thaler HT. Shorter symptom assessment instruments: the Condensed Memorial Symptom Assessment Scale (CMSAS). Cancer Invest. 2004;22(4):526–36. https://doi.org/10.1081/cnv-200026487.
26. Cleeland CS, Mendoza TR, Wang XS, Chou C, Harle MT, Morrissey M, Engstrom MC. Assessing symptom distress in cancer patients: the MD Anderson Symptom Inventory. Cancer. 2000;89(7):1634–46. https://doi.org/10.1002/1097-0142(20001001)89:7<1634::aid-cncr29>3.0.co;2-v.
27. de Haes JC, van Knippenberg FC, Neijt JP. Measuring psychological and physical distress in cancer patients: structure and application of the Rotterdam Symptom Checklist. Br J Cancer. 1990;62(6):1034–8. https://doi.org/10.1038/bjc.1990.434.
28. McCorkle R. The measurement of symptom distress. Semin Oncol Nurs. 1987;3(4):248–56. https://doi.org/10.1016/s0749-2081(87)80015-3.
29. Mystakidou K, Tsilika E, Parpa E, Katsouda E, Galanos A, Vlahos L. Psychological distress of patients with advanced cancer: influence and contribution of pain severity and pain interference. Cancer Nurs. 2006;29(5):400–5. https://doi.org/10.1097/00002820-200609000-00009.
30. Mitchell AJ, Chan M, Bhatti H, Halton M, Grassi L, Johansen C, Meader N. Prevalence of depression, anxiety, and adjustment disorder in oncological, haematological, and palliative-care settings: a meta-analysis of 94 interview-based studies. Lancet Oncol. 2011;12(2):160–74. https://doi.org/10.1016/S1470-2045(11)70002-X.
31. Block SD. Assessing and managing depression in the terminally ill patient. ACP–ASIM End-of-Life Care Consensus Panel. American College of Physicians–American Society of Internal Medicine. Ann Intern Med. 2000;132(3):209–18. https://doi.org/10.7326/0003-4819-132-3-200002010-00007.

32. Zung WW. A self-rating depression scale. Arch Gen Psychiatry. 1965;12:63–70. https://doi.org/10.1001/archpsyc.1965.01720310065008.
33. Satin JR, Linden W, Phillips MJ. Depression as a predictor of disease progression and mortality in cancer patients: a meta-analysis. Cancer. 2009;115(22):5349–61. https://doi.org/10.1002/cncr.24561.
34. Coyle N, Sculco L. Expressed desire for hastened death in seven patients living with advanced cancer: a phenomenologic inquiry. Oncol Nurs Forum. 2004;31(4):699–709. https://doi.org/10.1188/04.ONF.699-709.
35. Chochinov HM, Wilson KG, Enns M, Lander S. "Are you depressed?" Screening for depression in the terminally ill. Am J Psychiatry. 1997;154(5):674–6. https://doi.org/10.1176/ajp.154.5.674.
36. Mitchell AJ. Are one or two simple questions sufficient to detect depression in cancer and palliative care? A Bayesian meta-analysis. Br J Cancer. 2008;98(12):1934–43. https://doi.org/10.1038/sj.bjc.6604396.
37. Robinson S, Kissane DW, Brooker J, Burney S. A systematic review of the demoralization syndrome in individuals with progressive disease and cancer: a decade of research. J Pain Symptom Manage. 2015;49(3):595–610. https://doi.org/10.1016/j.jpainsymman.2014.07.008.
38. Robinson S, Kissane DW, Brooker J, Burney S. A review of the construct of demoralization: history, definitions, and future directions for palliative care. Am J Hosp Palliat Care. 2016;33(1):93–101. https://doi.org/10.1177/1049909114553461.
39. Tang PL, Wang HH, Chou FH. A systematic review and meta-analysis of demoralization and depression in patients with cancer. Psychosomatics. 2015;56(6):634–43. https://doi.org/10.1016/j.psym.2015.06.005.
40. Vehling S, Oechsle K, Koch U, Mehnert A. Receiving palliative treatment moderates the effect of age and gender on demoralization in patients with cancer. PLoS One. 2013;8(3):e59417. https://doi.org/10.1371/journal.pone.0059417.
41. Stark D, Kiely M, Smith A, Velikova G, House A, Selby P. Anxiety disorders in cancer patients: their nature, associations, and relation to quality of life. J Clin Oncol. 2002;20(14):3137–48. https://doi.org/10.1200/JCO.2002.08.549.
42. American Psychiatric Association. Diagnostic and statistical manual of mental disorders. 5th ed. Washington, DC: American Psychiatric Association; 2013.
43. Breitbart W, Alici Y. Evidence-based treatment of delirium in patients with cancer. J Clin Oncol. 2012;30(11):1206–14. https://doi.org/10.1200/JCO.2011.39.8784.
44. Fishman B, Pasternak S, Wallenstein SL, Houde RW, Holland JC, Foley KM. The Memorial Pain Assessment Card. A valid instrument for the evaluation of cancer pain. Cancer. 1987;60(5):1151–8. https://doi.org/10.1002/1097-0142(19870901)60:5<1151::aid-cncr2820600538>3.0.co;2-g.
45. Caraceni A, Nanni O, Maltoni M, Piva L, Indelli M, Arnoldi E, Monti M, Montanari L, Amadori D, De Conno F. Impact of delirium on the short term prognosis of advanced cancer patients. Italian Multicenter Study Group on Palliative Care. Cancer. 2000;89(5):1145–9. https://doi.org/10.1002/1097-0142(20000901)89:5<1145::aid-cncr24>3.0.co;2-x.
46. de la Cruz M, Ransing V, Yennu S, Wu J, Liu D, Reddy A, Delgado-Guay M, Bruera E. The frequency, characteristics, and outcomes among cancer patients with delirium admitted to an acute palliative care unit. Oncologist. 2015;20(12):1425–31. https://doi.org/10.1634/theoncologist.2015-0115.
47. Wada T, Wada M, Wada M, Onishi H. Characteristics, interventions, and outcomes of misdiagnosed delirium in cancer patients. Palliat Support Care. 2010;8(2):125–31. https://doi.org/10.1017/S1478951509990861.
48. Massie MJ, Miller K. Oncology. In: Levenson JL, editor. The American Psychiatric Publishing textbook of psychosomatic medicine: psychiatric care of the medically ill. 2nd ed. Washington, DC: American Psychiatric Publishing; 2011. p. 525–50.
49. Lawlor PG, Gagnon B, Mancini IL, Pereira JL, Hanson J, Suarez-Almazor ME, Bruera ED. Occurrence, causes, and outcome of delirium in patients with advanced cancer: a prospective study. Arch Intern Med. 2000;160(6):786–94. https://doi.org/10.1001/archinte.160.6.786.

50. Sarhill N, Walsh D, Nelson KA, LeGrand S, Davis MP. Assessment of delirium in advanced cancer: the use of the bedside confusion scale. Am J Hosp Palliat Care. 2001;18(5):335–41. https://doi.org/10.1177/104990910101800509.
51. Hudson PL, Remedios C, Thomas K. A systematic review of psychosocial interventions for family carers of palliative care patients. BMC Palliat Care. 2010;9:17. https://doi.org/10.1186/1472-684X-9-17.
52. Stewart AL, Teno J, Patrick DL, Lynn J. The concept of quality of life of dying persons in the context of health care. J Pain Symptom Manage. 1999;17(2):93–108. https://doi.org/10.1016/s0885-3924(98)00131-6.
53. Rocha SMM, Nascimento LC, de Lima RAG. Enfermagem pediátrica e abordagem da família: subsídios para o ensino de graduação [Pediatric nursing and the family approach: subsidies for undergraduate education]. Rev Lat Am Enfermagem. 2002;10(5):709–11. https://doi.org/10.1590/s0104-11692002000500013.
54. Franco MHP. A família em psico-oncologia [The family in psycho-oncology]. In: de Carvalho VA, MHP F, Kovács MJ, Liberato RP, Macieira RC, Veit MT, Gomes MJB, Barros LH, editors. Temas em psico-oncologia [Themes in psycho-oncology]. Sao Paulo: Summus; 2008. p. 358–61.
55. Leahey M, Wright LM. Enfermeiras e familias: um guia para avaliação e intervenção na família [Nurses and families: a guide to assessment and intervention in the family]. 3rd ed. Roca: Sao Paulo; 2002.
56. da Silva RCF, Hortale VA. Cuidados paliativos oncológicos: elementos para o debate de diretrizes nesta área [Palliative care in cancer: elements for debating the guidelines]. Cad Saude Publica. 2006;22(10):2055–66. https://doi.org/10.1590/S0102-311X2006001000011.
57. Sequeira CAC. Adaptação e validação da Escala de Sobrecarga do Cuidador de Zarit [Adaptation and validation of Zarit Burden Interview Scale]. Revista Referência. 2010;II(12):9–16.
58. Academia Nacional de Cuidados Paliativos. Manual de cuidados paliativos [Palliative care manual]. Rio de Janeiro: Diagraphic; 2009. p. 253–4.
59. Wolff JL, Dy SM, Frick KD, Kasper JD. End-of-life care: findings from a national survey of informal caregivers. Arch Intern Med. 2007;167(1):40–6. https://doi.org/10.1001/archinte.167.1.40.
60. Chari AV, Engberg J, Ray KN, Mehrotra A. The opportunity costs of informal elder-care in the United States: new estimates from the American Time Use Survey. Health Serv Res. 2015;50(3):871–82. https://doi.org/10.1111/1475-6773.12238.
61. Covinsky KE, Landefeld CS, Teno J, Connors AF Jr, Dawson N, Youngner S, Desbiens N, Lynn J, Fulkerson W, Reding D, Oye R, Phillips RS. Is economic hardship on the families of the seriously ill associated with patient and surrogate care preferences? SUPPORT Investigators. Arch Intern Med. 1996;156(15):1737–41.
62. Emanuel EJ, Fairclough DL, Emanuel LL. Attitudes and desires related to euthanasia and physician-assisted suicide among terminally ill patients and their caregivers. JAMA. 2000;284(19):2460–8. https://doi.org/10.1001/jama.284.19.2460.
63. Carvalho MCB, editor. A família contemporânea em debate [The contemporary family in debate]. Sao Paulo: EDUC/Cortez; 1995.
64. Vitale MAF. Famílias monoparentais: indagações [Single-parent families: questions]. Revista Serviço Social & Sociedade. 2002;XXIII(71):45–62.
65. Biffi RG, Mamede MV. Suporte social na reabilitação da mulher mastectomizada: o papel do parceiro sexual [Social support in the rehabilitation of mastectomized women: the role of the sexual partner]. Rev Esc Enferm USP. 2004;38(3):262–9. https://doi.org/10.1590/s0080-62342004000300004.
66. Swinton J. Spirituality in mental health care: rediscovering a 'forgotten' dimension. London: Jessica Kingsley; 2001.
67. Hay D, Nye R. The spirit of the child. London: Jessica Kingsley; 2006.
68. Anderson RS. Spiritual caregiving as secular sacrament: a practical theology for professional caregivers. London: Jessica Kingsley; 2003.

69. Tervalon M, Murray-García J. Cultural humility versus cultural competence: a critical distinction in defining physician training outcomes in multicultural education. J Health Care Poor Underserved. 1998;9(2):117–25. https://doi.org/10.1353/hpu.2010.0233.
70. Campinha-Bacote J. The process of cultural competence in the delivery of healthcare services: a model of care. J Transcult Nurs. 2002;13(3):181–201. https://doi.org/10.1177/10459602013003003.
71. Ferrell BR, Twaddle ML, Melnick A, Meier DE. National consensus project clinical practice guidelines for quality palliative care guidelines, 4th edition. J Palliat Med. 2018;21(12):1684–9. https://doi.org/10.1089/jpm.2018.0431.
72. Koenig BA, Gates-Williams J. Understanding cultural difference in caring for dying patients. West J Med. 1995;163(3):244–9.
73. Taylor JS. Confronting "culture" in medicine's "culture of no culture". Acad Med. 2003;78(6):555–9. https://doi.org/10.1097/00001888-200306000-00003.
74. Kim EK. "A word can become a seed": a lesson learned about cultural humility. J Cancer Educ. 2016;31(4):813–5. https://doi.org/10.1007/s13187-015-0878-0.
75. Foronda C, Baptiste DL, Reinholdt MM, Ousman K. Cultural humility: a concept analysis. J Transcult Nurs. 2016;27(3):210–7. https://doi.org/10.1177/1043659615592677.
76. Sanders JJ, Robinson MT, Block SD. Factors impacting advance care planning among African Americans: results of a systematic integrated review. J Palliat Med. 2016;19(2):202–27. https://doi.org/10.1089/jpm.2015.0325.
77. Chochinov HM, McClement S, Hack T, Thompson G, Dufault B, Harlos M. Eliciting personhood within clinical practice: effects on patients, families, and health care providers. J Pain Symptom Manage. 2015;49(6):974–980.e2. https://doi.org/10.1016/j.jpainsymman.2014.11.291.
78. Phelps AC, Maciejewski PK, Nilsson M, Balboni TA, Wright AA, Paulk ME, Trice E, Schrag D, Peteet JR, Block SD, Prigerson HG. Religious coping and use of intensive life-prolonging care near death in patients with advanced cancer. JAMA. 2009;301(11):1140–7. https://doi.org/10.1001/jama.2009.341.
79. Rodin D, Balboni M, Mitchell C, Smith PT, VanderWeele TJ, Balboni TA. Whose role? Oncology practitioners' perceptions of their role in providing spiritual care to advanced cancer patients. Support Care Cancer. 2015;23(9):2543–50. https://doi.org/10.1007/s00520-015-2611-2.
80. Zhang B, Nilsson ME, Prigerson HG. Factors important to patients' quality of life at the end of life. Arch Intern Med. 2012;172(15):1133–42. https://doi.org/10.1001/archinternmed.2012.2364.
81. Balboni TA, Vanderwerker LC, Block SD, Paulk ME, Lathan CS, Peteet JR, Prigerson HG. Religiousness and spiritual support among advanced cancer patients and associations with end-of-life treatment preferences and quality of life. J Clin Oncol. 2007;25(5):555–60. https://doi.org/10.1200/JCO.2006.07.9046.
82. Balboni TA, Balboni M, Enzinger AC, Gallivan K, Paulk ME, Wright A, Steinhauser K, VanderWeele TJ, Prigerson HG. Provision of spiritual support to patients with advanced cancer by religious communities and associations with medical care at the end of life. JAMA Intern Med. 2013;173(12):1109–17. https://doi.org/10.1001/jamainternmed.2013.903.
83. Steinhauser KE, Voils CI, Clipp EC, Bosworth HB, Christakis NA, Tulsky JA. "Are you at peace?": one item to probe spiritual concerns at the end of life. Arch Intern Med. 2006;166(1):101–5. https://doi.org/10.1001/archinte.166.1.101.
84. Chochinov HM, Hack T, Hassard T, Kristjanson LJ, McClement S, Harlos M. Dignity therapy: a novel psychotherapeutic intervention for patients near the end of life. J Clin Oncol. 2005;23(24):5520–5. https://doi.org/10.1200/JCO.2005.08.391.
85. Smith-Stoner M. End-of-life preferences for atheists. J Palliat Med. 2007;10(4):923–8. https://doi.org/10.1089/jpm.2006.0197.

Chapter 7
Practical Considerations in End-of-Life Care

The process of dying is one of medicine's greatest mysteries. We are still not able to identify precisely which are the mechanisms that initiate the process of dying and after which moment it really becomes irreversible. However, despite all of the advances and the commitment of science to life, few health professionals, especially physicians, acquire expertise in the technical and emotional knowledge necessary for the care of the dying person. Within the process of dying, there is still plenty of space for life.

Palliative care has become a symbol of close death, since it is only in the last moments that the reality of "having nothing else to do" is considered. This is why the stigma of palliative care is so deep and painful.

Despite the reach of the palliative care approach throughout the course of a serious, incurable, and uncontrollable illness, most patients in Brazil—if they are admitted to palliative care—will receive its benefits only at the very end.

7.1 Concepts

From a conceptual point of view, a terminally ill patient is one with a short life expectancy. In the USA and Europe, a candidate for palliative care is a patient whose life expectancy is ≤ 6 months, as attested by two physicians. Prognostic data need to be constantly reviewed and supported by knowledge of which stage of the disease's evolution the patient is at and also their functional compromise [1]. Clinical conditions concerning comorbidities and the functional impact of life-lengthening treatment that can still be offered to the patient must also be taken into consideration.

A. C. L. Q. Arantes, *Clinical Assessment of Human Suffering*,
https://doi.org/10.1007/978-3-030-57535-9_7

7.2 The Last Weeks of Life

In the situation of a disease with a faster evolution, such as cancer, the patient starts to present a more significant functional decline, becoming more dependent in the activities of daily life and often developing a need for self-care assistance. In chronic situations—such as dementia, heart failure, chronic pulmonary disease, and permanent neurological conditions—the patient already presents signs of major compromise, which may result in repeated infections, severe malnutrition, and pressure ulcers.

When clinical events become frequent, with a new situation of irreversible frailty, the patient may be facing a life expectancy measured in weeks. At this time, it is really important that the conversation about anticipated directives for life support be re-evaluated with the family and, whenever possible, also with the patient. Orientations concerning the current process and its dynamics, as well as the availability of the doctor and the care team in the face of these oscillations, become true priorities for the family and the patient.

7.3 The Last Days of Life

To maintain the serenity of the patient, the family, and the team in the last days of a person's life, it is very valuable for the physician to be familiar with the physiological changes that occur in the process of dying. Death may be easily diagnosed, but the process that is initiated and that runs until the death event happens can be long and frightening. When it depends on the ability of the physician to manage this moment of finitude, we can think of a delicate but serene period or one full of tensions, futile procedures, and more suffering both for the patient and for their family. Increases in weakness and fatigue, and diminutions in appetite and liquid ingestion, can be expected.

Consequently, we will observe decreased peripheral perfusion, neurological dysfunction, the possibility of manifestation of pain, and loss of ability to close the eyes. Because of the worsening of weakness and fatigue, the patient has a decreased ability to move by themselves, with an increased risk of pressure ulcers and a need for greater care. The decreases in appetite and water ingestion may lead the family to manifest anxiety and dread of the myth of the patient "dying from hunger and thirst"; at this moment, it is important to remind oneself (because this conversation needs to have been had at earlier stages) that at this stage, food can be nauseating for the patient and anorexia can be a protective mechanism against the risk of bronchoaspiration [2].

7.4 The Last Hours of Life

The quality of time at this stage of human life seems to be dilated. This may mean that a few hours are perceived as long days. At this moment, it is important to seek to offer the patient and their family all of the privacy and intimacy that is possible, but with no connotation of abandonment.

Hence, it is very important to show commitment and special attention in ensuring comfort, maintenance of the patient's routine care, and continuation of the medication prescribed for the management of pain and other symptoms. Review of medical and nursing prescriptions at this stage is aimed at maintaining the essentials for the patient's comfort and avoiding use of measures that are unnecessary for their well-being (Fig. 7.1).

In the event that this period occurs in the patient's home, foreseeing the need for special equipment (such as a hospital bed, aspirator, drip, intravenous medication, and diapers) is recommended. Consider alternative access routes for medication when the patient can no longer swallow or is unconscious.

In home assistance, it is fundamental to maintain regularity in the re-evaluation of the care plan.

7.5 Preparing People for the Process of Dying

This is one of the most precious stages of palliative care: preparation in the face of the process of dying. With regard to direct caregivers and closest relatives, it is very important to be aware of the patient's choices, demonstrating confidence in the information offered, commitment, and empathy, with quick responses to requests. Early orientation to the signs and physiological changes expected at this stage of care helps families find alternatives to offer care.

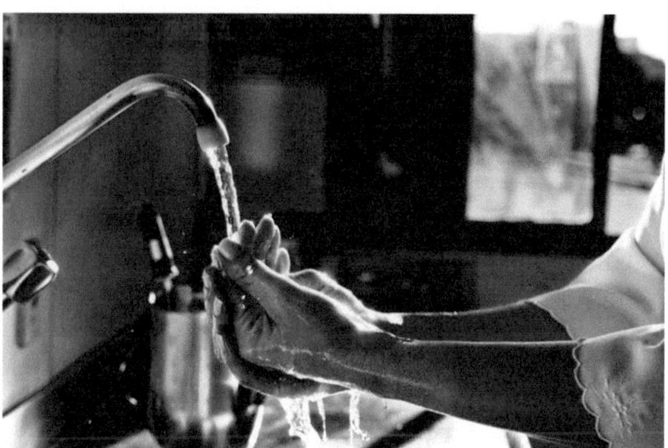

Fig. 7.1 In the last moments of life, it is very important to show commitment and special attention in ensuring comfort and maintenance of the patient's routine care

Keeping the patient subhydrated may be more comfortable for them, as it spares the need for frequent diaper changes and decreases sweating, physiological secretions from airways, and gastrointestinal fluids. This is why plenty of caution is required to avoid excessive administration of fluids via the parenteral route. Consequently, it is necessary to double care for the mucosae and dry eye syndrome; local lubrication is indicated and provides greater comfort.

In the last hours, we can observe a more significant decrease in blood perfusion, tachycardia, hypotension, cold extremities, cyanosis, a skin rash, and a decrease in urine volume. It is worth noting that at this stage, prescription of parenteral fluids does not revert this picture!

In relation to the progression of neurological dysfunction, the patient may present a spontaneous decrease in their consciousness level. At these moments, it becomes a challenge to maintain communication with the patient, leading to an increase in the family's anxiety. Therefore, in orientation, assume that the patient can hear anything, reinforce the importance of talking to them and conveying safety and presence, and, as soon as possible, encourage the patient's relatives and closest friends to verbalize permission to die. In situations where the patient appears to develop agitation with manifestation of great discomfort, a discussion about palliative sedation is suitable.

7.6 Palliative Sedation

Palliative sedation is a specialized procedure intended to control symptoms of intense suffering that are refractory to conventional treatment. It is defined as medically induced lowering of the consciousness level in patients who present severe, untreatable, or refractory symptoms, with attention to pain, dyspnea, asthenia, anorexia, confusion, and massive hemorrhage. For prescription of palliative sedation, we must be sure that this is the only way to ensure the patient's comfort [3–5].

The first point to be discussed is the patient's and their family's agreement prior to this procedure. In the event that it is not possible to obtain the patient's consent, the family establishes this decision with the doctor ALWAYS on the basis of the patient's comfort. It is not justified to prescribe sedation for patients because they have no prognosis, because "no prognosis" is not a refractory symptom.

The second point is the choice of the medication to be utilized. *Sedation* is obtained by the administration of *sedatives*; therefore, using opiates with the objective of sedating a patient is wrong. Unless the patient presents an appearance of intense pain or severe dyspnea, the use of opiates is not indicated. The practice of prescribing "M1" solution (pethidine, chlorpromazine, and promethazine) is also inadequate, since the pethidine used in this solution (through its metabolite norpethidine) promotes intoxication of the central nervous system, leading to agitation and increasing the risk of respiratory depression and seizures a few hours after its continued use. It is fundamental to reinforce the fact that palliative care aims to alleviate suffering and not to abbreviate the life of the sufferer.

7.7 When Death Happens

In the absence of a pulse, heartbeat, and breathing movements, the presence of dilated and fixed pupils, a drop in body temperature, waxlike skin paleness, and relaxation of muscles and sphincters are signs that death has occurred. There may be releases of feces and urine, the eyes may remain open, and the jaw drops.

All of these details should have been explained to the family and direct caregivers during the process prior to the patient's death, especially in situations where a home death has been chosen. These orientations are very precious in maintaining the calm of everyone around the patient, especially when death occurs in the absence of a certified health professional to attest to it.

7.8 What Not to Do When a Natural Death Happens

When the whole process of finitude has been supported under the palliative care perspective, and the family and the patient agree to the acceptance of a natural death, then when death is attested, it is necessary to maintain the order of the moment:

- Do not call the emergency services.
- Do not try to revive the patient.
- Have a list ready of people who must be called.
- Verify if there is an expressed desire for organ donation.
- Continue to reinforce the importance of religious or cultural rites.

Be aware that loss is felt in different ways by each of those who stay—and respect each of their expressions! Allow the necessary time to witness what has happened, creating a peaceful environment accessible to all who desire to get closer, and ensuring support for acute reactions of suffering for the loss.

7.9 Care of the Body After Death

- Prepare the body according to the traditions allowed by the family.
- Maintain support for the funeral preparations.
- Notify the other physicians and professionals involved in the patient's care.
  - Stop the patient's medication.
  - Remove the supplies and equipment.
  - Remove the medication and materials used (gloves, gauze, etc.).

7.10 Planning of Grief Support

Establish a plan of action, together with the family, for the grief period. The planning of a meeting with the team involved in the patient's care, so that everyone can express their experience and their suffering before the loss, can be a very significant experience for everyone involved, including the assistance team.

And the next day . . .
Life goes on . . .
different, but following its course . . .
always different.

References

1. World Health Organization. Symptom relief in terminal illness. Geneva: World Health Organization; 1998. https://apps.who.int/iris/handle/10665/42121. Accessed 10 Aug 2020.
2. de Simone G, Tripodoro V. Fundamentos de cuidados paliativos y control de sintomas [Fundamentals of palliative care and symptom control]. Buenos Aires: Pallium; 2004. https://www.pallium.com.ar/wp-content/uploads/2019/10/FUNDAMENTOS-DE-CUIDADOS-PALIATIVOS-y-control-de-sintomas.pdf. Accessed .
3. Doyle D, Hanks GW, MacDonald N, editors. Oxford textbook of palliative medicine. 2nd ed. New York: Oxford University Press; 1999.
4. Jeroen G, Hasselaar J, et al. Improving prescription in palliative sedation compliance with Dutch guidelines. 2nd ed. Oxford: Oxford University Press; 1998.
5. Vissers KC, Hasselaar J, Verhagen SA. Sedation in palliative care. Curr Opin Anaesthesiol. 2007;20(2):137–42. https://doi.org/10.1097/ACO.0b013e328049557b.

Chapter 8
Grief and Bereavement: Practical Considerations for Health Professionals

8.1 Anticipatory Grief

Anticipatory grief is the experience of each of the stages of mourning experienced by the patient and their loved ones during the illness process, where the awareness of finitude happens. Being aware of your death means that the entire grieving process is experienced in advance as a perception of the reality of the death that will come. Mourning is the social manifestation of a socially assumed feeling of grief in the face of an experience of loss. Our life is inevitably forever affected by the end of a relationship, situation, project, or dream.

The most common reactions to the grieving experience can be emotional, physical, cognitive, and behavioral in nature, and can last for a variable time—maybe just a few days, or even a few months. Feelings may include shock, sadness, guilt, anger and hostility, loneliness, agitation, anxiety, fatigue, longing (a desire to be with the deceased person), helplessness, and relief. They may be accompanied by physical sensations, which are generally described as a pit in the stomach, tightness in the chest, a lump in the throat, hypersensitivity to noise, a feeling of depersonalization ("I walk on the street and there is no real world, including me"), shortness of breath, muscle weakness, lack of energy, a dry mouth, somatic complaints, and susceptibility to diseases (especially diseases linked to low immunity, stress, or lack of health care).

From a cognitive point of view, the experience of loss can lead to disbelief, confusion, memory and concentration deficits, obsessive thoughts, the sensation of a presence, or hallucinations. Changes in the grieving person's social behavior are manifested through sleep disturbance; a loss/increase in appetite; increased consumption of psychotropics, alcohol, and tobacco; "aerial" behavior; social isolation; avoidance of things that remind them of the person who died; searching and calling for the person; dreams about the deceased; hyperactivity; and restlessness.

The family lives an extremely disturbing experience throughout the patient's end-of-life trajectory, not only because of the physical and emotional stress inherent

A. C. L. Q. Arantes, *Clinical Assessment of Human Suffering*,
https://doi.org/10.1007/978-3-030-57535-9_8

in the provision of care but also because of feelings of loss and separation caused by the patient's illness and imminent death [1–3]. However, this experience is considered a necessary and significant part of the process of adaptation prior to the loss [4, 5]. Lindemann [6] coined the term *anticipatory grief* (AG) to describe grief expressed in advance when a loss is threatened or inevitable, and it refers to any such suffering experienced by the patient or by a survivor before the death occurs [7]. Anticipatory grief can then be assessed as a continuous and irreversible process, analogous to the necessary adjustment in the period that happens after death. Family caregivers are a key component in palliative care, and anticipatory grief issues are considered of particular concern.

Elisabeth Kübler-Ross's book *On Death and Dying* [8] sparked widespread academic and popular interest in the emotional scene of death. Its publication in 1969 also coincided, roughly, with two important developments that have changed the way in which patients die and their loved ones experience the process of their death: first, the widespread rejection of medical paternalism in favor of decision-making models that prioritize the patient's autonomy; and second, the increasing prevalence of chronic diseases (cancer, mainly) that extend the process of dying and often lead to long periods when patients are unable to make decisions. Together, these two developments have helped to create clinical environments in which health care surrogates (often members of the dying individual's family) play an increasing role in end-of-life choices.

On Death and Dying was conceived as an exploration of dying from the perspective of dying patients, but it was later reused and served as the basis for the theory of the five stages of mourning. Surprisingly, very little subsequent research in bioethics has explored the specifics of the connection between grief and clinical decision making on the part of doctors acting as patients' health care surrogates. The standard logic for the use of health care surrogates is that an appropriate surrogate's choice can honor the patient's autonomy because—thanks to the surrogate's understanding of the values or preferences of the dying patient—surely they can choose the courses of treatment that the noncompetent patient would have chosen had they been competent to make a choice. However, doctors' surrogate decisions routinely fail to meet this "substituted judgment" standard. Instead of focusing on the perceived values and preferences of the dying patient, many surrogates adopt a decision-making approach that can be charitably described as "multifaceted" [9], recognizing that their surrogate choices are shaped by their own treatment preferences, spiritual beliefs, or experiences that they are supposed to have in common with the patient [10].

Not everyone dies as a result of a chronic disease. Sometimes, death comes suddenly. People can die on the operating table, in a plane accident, in a car, in an assault, or in a hospital emergency room. In this context, sudden death is an important risk factor for complication of the grieving experience. This can also happen when family members and caregivers do not accept the possibility that a serious illness or condition can be fatal and are not expecting the patient's death when it happens.

The health effects of the mourning period—and even the risk of mortality in the most vulnerable people, such as the elderly—are well known and documented.

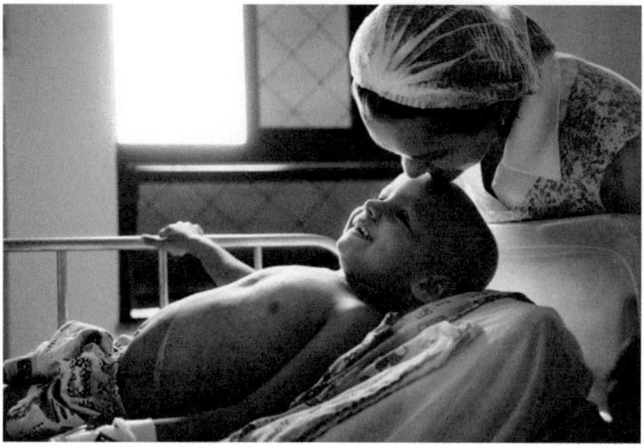

Fig. 8.1 Kindness is necessary for a healthy grieving process in an experience of loss

Although the evidence is clear, little or nothing is done to minimize the risk of life-threatening problems in people in the grieving process. It is very important to remember that grieving is an intense and necessary process, but that caring for the health of the grieving person, in all of its dimensions, is essential for the pain to go away and leave only the memory of what was lived, with even greater value (Fig. 8.1).

References

1. Waldrop DP, Kramer BJ, Skretny JA, Milch RA, Finn W. Final transitions: family caregiving at the end of life. J Palliat Med. 2005;8(3):623–38. https://doi.org/10.1089/jpm.2005.8.623.
2. Given B, Wyatt G, Given C, Sherwood P, Gift A, DeVoss D, Rahbar M. Burden and depression among caregivers of patients with cancer at the end of life. Oncol Nurs Forum. 2004;31(6):1105–17. https://doi.org/10.1188/04.ONF.1105-1117.
3. Sales E. Family burden and quality of life. Qual Life Res. 2003;12 Suppl 1:33–41. https://doi.org/10.1023/a:1023513218433.
4. Hebert RS, Dang Q, Schulz R. Preparedness for the death of a loved one and mental health in bereaved caregivers of patients with dementia: findings from the REACH study. J Palliat Med. 2006;9(3):683–93. https://doi.org/10.1089/jpm.2006.9.683.
5. Hebert RS, Schulz R, Copeland VC, Arnold RM. Preparing family caregivers for death and bereavement: insights from caregivers of terminally ill patients. J Pain Symptom Manage. 2009;37(1):3–12. https://doi.org/10.1016/j.jpainsymman.2007.12.010.
6. Lindemann E. Symptomatology and management of acute grief. Am J Psychiatry. 1994;151(6 Suppl):155–60. https://doi.org/10.1176/ajp.151.6.155.
7. Aldrich CK. Some dynamics of anticipatory grief. In: Schoenberg B, Carr AC, Peretz D, Kutscher AH, editors. Anticipatory grief. New York: Columbia University Press; 1974. p. 3–9.
8. Kübler-Ross E. On death and dying. New York: Scribner; 1969.
9. Li L, Nelson JE, Hanson LC, Cox CE, Carson SS, Chai EJ, Keller KL, Tulsky JA, Danis M. How surrogate decision-makers for patients with chronic critical illness perceive and carry out their role. Crit Care Med. 2018;46(5):699–704. https://doi.org/10.1097/CCM.0000000000003035.
10. Fritsch J, Petronio S, Helft PR, Torke AM. Making decisions for hospitalized older adults: ethical factors considered by family surrogates. J Clin Ethics. 2013;24(2):125–34.

Chapter 9
Accomplishments, Unfinished Business, and Regrets

Looking back, in the face of finitude, is what brings the greatest unrest. When faced with the consciousness of death, the first thing we look at is the life we have had up until that moment. The time comes to rethink the choices made a long time ago—that moment when you think, "Have I taken the right path? Had I taken the longest path, would it have been nicer and taken longer to arrive?"

The first question is: what if there were a way of you not being there? This is the first questioning. "Oh, if only I hadn't smoked, I wouldn't have lung cancer!" or "If I hadn't drunk and driven, I wouldn't be here!" or "If I hadn't lived so inadequately, I wouldn't have clogged coronary arteries now!" or "If I hadn't been born into this family, I wouldn't have this disease!" When you have time, you can go back and make a new choice, for regret supposes that you can come around, make a U-turn, and instead follow the path you consider to be the right one. But in the time of regret, it is always the classic "You have made a mistake, and you are doomed. The problem is that when you made that choice you now deem wrong, you did not even realize you were going the wrong way."

An Australian nurse, Bronnie Ware [1], worked with patients in their final life stages, who were known as "terminal" patients. She made house calls and started to notice that during the conversations she had the opportunity of having with these dying people, there were some recurring themes linked to regret. Her experiences inspired the writing of her book *The Top Five Regrets of the Dying*. She was very insightful in proposing these five aspects, and she was actually right, because I see this happen in my patients day by day. One of these regrets is "I wish I had made more of my choices instead of making choices to please others." When we talk about this, I think a lot of people regret the same thing. And when the end comes, what you want as payment for your wasted lifetime is all of the time you gave to another, doing things you believed were good for another. However, no one asked you for anything. You did it because you wanted to, for the noblest or the most selfish of reasons. But most of the times when you did something to please someone else, you did it because you believed that person would be happy if you did it. Between the lines, you were making a choice to validate your importance in another

A. C. L. Q. Arantes, *Clinical Assessment of Human Suffering*,
https://doi.org/10.1007/978-3-030-57535-9_9

person's life. Using your time of living to become important in someone else's life is a very crooked path of existence. If you can be yourself and be loved for that reason alone, then consider yourself a happy human being. But if you need to become someone else to consider yourself loved, then there is something wrong going on. Much regret will come later. It is a very dangerous path—wanting to be someone based on what you represent to another. Going back to that situation of helping someone to die, understand this: that person is not dying for you to feel useful.

That is not the goal. You are not there to make sure you are any good. Being in your place beside someone who is dying is much larger than your existence. Your existence exists for you to exist; it is as simple as breathing. But throughout our lives, we start conditioning our decisions to be favorable to others. We "subcontract" the beneficiaries of our decisions. We direct the results of our decisions in favor of people who have not asked us to make that choice. "Oh, I am going to work a lot because I want to give my children all of this," or "I will not eat; I will not sleep; I will work from sunrise to sunset so I can afford to send them to a very expensive school, so they can be doctors and engineers and lawyers." Yet the child wants to be an artist, wants to travel and see the world. And you do not bother to value and believe in the capacity for decision making that your child might have. You do not bother to believe that you can talk to them and clarify the paths both of you can take toward a truer choice.

The answer in relation to our frustrations comes as outrage. "How come?" or "I have sacrificed so much for you!" or "How ungrateful!" And there are reactions that are terrible to experience. I had the opportunity to care for a senior lady with advanced dementia, who experienced over 20 years of bedridden dependence. Her daughter yelled that her mother could not die: "I gave my life for her! When I was 20, my wedding date was set, the invitations had been sent, the church was ready, everything had been paid for, and then she said to me, 'Are you going to abandon me when I am old and sick?'" And this daughter left everything behind, canceled her wedding, and left school to take care of her mother.

And then 35 years passed. How come her mother was now dying—by what right? What was she to do with the rest of her life after she had given the best part of it to her mother? Of course, for her, her mother could not die. "Treat her, give her morphine because she cannot die . . . intubate her, do all you can, because she has to live. My life depends on it."

This story is a dramatic story, an extreme of suffering. When the mother demanded that her daughter abandon her own life, her daughter did not know how to say that she could take care of her in a different way. She fell for the emotional blackmail and regretted it. But her regret came too late and became a lament. It was already the point of no return.

How many times throughout our lives do we interpret the same requests and abdicate from living our lives on the basis of an expectation someone else has of us?

We keep collecting moments in life when we make decisions to please someone else, and we will end our days on the basis of these choices. Something that occurs very frequently in hospitals and seniors' clinics is severe criticism of "abandonment" of people on their deathbeds. But it is very important not to pass judgment concerning a patient's solitude in a hospital. People think that because a person has cancer or is over 60 years old, they suddenly became saints, worthy of being idolized and loved by the entire family. That is not how life works. We cultivate the quality of our relationships, and it is on the basis of this cultivation that we will enjoy good company or no company at the end of life. How does this abandonment happen? Who is that person who is in the hospital? When thinking about our regrets, who will we be in the hospital? Will we be an immense bottomless pit who has only given, given, given, but never received?

And then, if you are an empty pit, empty you will remain. It is going to be very difficult to rebuild relationships and live meaningful stories after completing such a long, hard, and concretely cruel path. It is possible that, in the end, you will be able to build a relationship with the health professionals who are caring for you. Many people die receiving love from their caregivers. It is very common that people in the hospital, even those who have had very complex relationships, end up making very beautiful bonds with us. In this moment, in which you realize that you have made decisions in favor of other people's joy and happiness—and that they have not asked for it and are not happy with the decisions you have made—regret comes and hurts too much. That is a pain no morphine can soothe.

Another regret concerns whether you could have expressed your emotions better. In Ware's book [1], she talks about "demonstrating love," but if you contextualize all of the stories she reports, she is talking about expressing emotions expressing what you are really feeling, even if such emotions are considered bad.

Throughout our process of growing, of education, we learn to control the expression of our emotions through control and commitment, as though we are wearing a mask—a cover. And in order to be accepted, to be heard, to be understood, we are capable of hiding much of what we feel. We believe that not demonstrating feelings can protect us throughout life. Experimenting in relationships, throughout our lives, puts us in certain situations in which we feel great pain, and we start defending ourselves from feeling pain again. "I did this and got hurt," or "Someone did this to me and I was hurt," and "There is no way am I going to do this," or "I don't want it to happen again."

And, in a silly way, we act as if all of the people who would cross our path were clones of the first person who hurt us. We have a tendency to believe that everyone is the same. There are people who think everybody is getting paid to do them harm. That is not so. There is no such possibility; not everyone is your enemy.

Everyone just wants to be happy. Even those people who do you harm also want the same thing as you: to be happy. This is maybe the greatest idea of freedom that Buddhist philosophy has brought me: everyone wants to be happy. And it is this desire that the best and the worst human beings have in common with me. I have learned that there is no one in the world who was born only to make me unhappy. When you are afraid of showing yourself, you do not say what you are feeling; you wear a mask.

Throughout our lives, we start collecting masks, and we wear the masks that better fit our style. If you want to be accepted, you put on the nice, thoughtful, polite mask, always being ready to help, always wanted, always wonderful; everyone can count on you; everyone adores you. And then the moment comes when you take off the mask and everyone sees you. Naked in body and soul. And if you were good only in order to please, then you will understand that you need to be really good in order to face the solitude at the end of life. In some way, the truth always surfaces throughout your relationships; if you continue being untrue but think you are being true, the other person ends up noticing it. And then you are alone in the story, and there are many stories like that in the hospital—stories of people who helped many others and now find themselves alone there. But they have managed to reach a single goal: feeling safe.

It is not the relationships they have built. The search for safety within affection is a black hole. You may find anything but true affection. You wear the mask of good relations and, in the end, what you find is the back of your mask. In the end, we learn to control the expression of our emotions through control and commitment, as though we are wearing a mask—a cover. You kept the other person from entering a great volcano of transformation. Meeting with another is what transforms you. Meeting with your own expectations, with your own reflections—in self-help books, in lectures, and in everything else—is no good without another. The inner world does not offer great potential for transformation; what does is true engagement with another, because it is from another human being that we receive the keys to some doors that are locked within us and that keep great revelations and secrets about us. I may have the key to open your heart. I may have the key to open your heart in the section of anger.

When you look at me, all you can think is how insufferable I am. Thus, it is not pleasant meeting me, because you feel anger. There are other people who open spaces inside you that reveal love, peace, joy. This means that I have the key that opens the little door that says love, peace, joy in your heart. I cannot bring you anything you do not already have. Many authors, writers, and thinkers have said that, but the most amazing thing is witnessing it happening before our eyes, in our hearts. I can bring you something you still do not know you possess. To me, this is very clear when I face the deaths of those I care for. I know that all of this essence of consciousness of death exists, so I know that it is within everyone. If I can open the right door, everyone will find the same thing as I did. The expression of affection is what transforms, and you feel fulfilled in life if you have been the instrument of transformation.

With regard to relationships of affection—whether these be considered good or not-so-good affections—making value judgments about what we feel can be very dangerous in the final moments: "This is good to feel," or This is not good to feel." It can be terrible realizing what you really feel in times like these. "Should I wish for my mother's death!?" or "Can I feel hatred for my father!?" or "Do I want this person, whom I'm supposed to love so much, to die?" This thought crosses the mind; it surfaces because it has no control. Emotion comes spontaneously, and through thought, you try to select and decide in your conscience if it is good or bad, and whether you are allowed to feel it or not.

So people believe that demonstrating good affection is nice, beautiful, and friendly, and that demonstrating bad affection is neither nice, nor beautiful, nor friendly. However, often it is through bad affection that we really transform. We are not always able to reach people, or to be reached, through the gentle path of joy. It is possible—and I am not saying that suffering is the only way—but it is very possible that suffering has an undeniable capacity to transform. What is the great drama we have here? "I feel hurt by most people here, but no one knows," or "I am very angry at you, but I will not tell you that," or "I don't want to speak because I can't; I don't deal well with conflict." What happens when you do not express affection is that this affection stays within you.

The energy of affection does not dissipate, especially when these feelings come from close relationships. The process of trying to cure bad feelings—internal recycling—generates toxic residue, and often we do not realize it. The strongest healing process possible is honest expression of what we feel.

Also, there is the understanding that having enemies is not all bad. Sometimes it is through them that we find strength and overpowering courage. Our friends love us the way we are. We believe we will give our friends the best, but for many people, it is their enemies who demand their best. We want to be happier, stronger, more successful, more everything. In the face of our enemies, we must demonstrate unbelievable strength. These conflict situations make us face difficult feelings, and people who do us apparent harm can be a great source of transformation for the best, for us to discover a force within us—our might. I do not speak about vengeance, but about a capacity to appropriate a force to demonstrate how much you can handle. In this demonstration of affection, even when it is demonstrating affection that is hard to deal with, you are verbalizing and giving the other person in front of you the opportunity to transform.

There, in this process, you also have to be open in order to transform yourself. You have to feel the pain of opening up so you can heal the soul sealed inside resentment. Only those who have survived have scars; the ones who left their wound open died miserably. Then the end of the road comes, in front of the final wall, and you regret not having demonstrated affection for people who may not exist anymore—the matter of regretting not having told your father you loved him, or your mother, your son, or your wife. These moments when we have lost the chance to demonstrate what we are actually feeling surface at full throttle at the end of life. But when this happens and it is with a living person, and there is a way for you to call, to meet again . . . and you do it . . . oh, it is beautiful to live this!

Another regret is having worked too hard. For many people, we are always working too hard. I feel that if you have a job that gives you the chance to make the world different, for the better, and you are involved in this work with this energy of transformation and are fulfilled, you see and feel meaning in the flow you have chosen to live. We have people who live with a tendency to treat life as something feasible, where you do things. There are people who believe living is having things, and they work like crazy to have, to hoard—hoarding not only material possessions but also resentments and crises. They may have many things, including problems.

The considerations I notice from this daily process that may cause regret happen when you need a mask to survive within the workplace. When there is a difference between who you are in your personal life and who you are at work, then you are in serious trouble.

You look at a scene and cannot recognize yourself, but you know how to justify it: that person there at work is a different being, who is there to do that job; I am another person. This distancing is what makes you think you are sacrificing your life in favor of another moment. Because you are far away, you are not there inside that lab coat, that suit, that tie, that plan. If you know how to be yourself only when wearing flip-flops, then put your feet on the ground before it is too late and before you no longer know the difference between your skin and the soles of your shoes. It is not only people who work in a business suit, a fancy dress, a company uniform, or a lab coat who are unhappy. There are many people who work in art, or who work in the creative world, who are completely unhappy.

We all have judgments concerning the work of others, but each of us knows the weight of the burden we bear. There are people who always think the life of another is always better, but that is not always true. This matter of positioning yourself at work in a way that is distanced from your essence will give you the feeling that you have wasted time, especially if you enjoy your essence better than your work. But there is also a risk when you enjoy better who you are at work—if you think you are someone only because you work. These people may be amazing at work, but in their personal lives, they are a disaster. And when they retire, it is as if they have died. They play a part in a much more fluid way in their workplace than in their own lives.

This happens very frequently with health professionals. These people are often completely unhappy in their personal lives because they work in health care. This has to do with that thing of being useful, giving, caring. It has the universal recommendation of doing unto others as you would have them do unto you. But most of the time, among health professionals and people who like to help and care for others, it is something very unhealthy. They do for other people what they cannot do for themselves. This is a very bad rule. "At my work, there is a mother losing a child; why would I complain about my life? Her life is much worse than mine." This tendency of the health professional, the savior, the caregiver, the volunteer—people who have a tendency of choosing a life of work that is related to helping others—is very complicated because during this process of working for others, they do not meet the other; they only give. There is a barrier in their genuine relationship with another. As a health professional, you are present in another person's life, wearing a fairy godmother mask; you only give and do not let yourself receive. This attitude makes you miss the chance to truly know the person you are caring for and makes you feel drained at the end of the day. However, when you do this work with your presence and open up to the possibility of exchange of learning and transformation, you feel renewed at the end of the day. At times, I end my day tired by the hours I work, leaving home at 6 o'clock and often not returning until after 11 p.m. But my energy tends to always stay high, and I am always whole. I get physically tired, like everyone in the process of commuting in the city of Sao Paulo, through hours of traffic, with doubled attention for fear of violence. But caring, working, doing things for others, and remaining available for another to transform me never makes me tired. I get tired only on days when I do not feel like opening up: "Not today; it's hard opening up." And when I realize that, I clear my schedule. If I cannot be present with another, if I need moments in which it is necessary to connect with myself, I am at peace with this decision.

Therapy, meditation, art, or poetry—doing anything that may connect me with the essence of who I am—teaches me and makes me understand that it is possible to be absolutely sure that the world goes round even though I am not pushing it. This is a challenge for those who are caregivers, who think things will only come out right if they are in control. These people, when they reach the end of life, feel that life owes them something. The matter of work permeates this crisis, but why, after all? How much of our lives do we spend at work? Most of us spend at least 8 hours at work each day. We are around for 30% of the time, work for 30%, and spend 30% doing things to try to improve our work performance. You meditate to have more attention, and you do more physical activity to be able to feel better physically—all for you to work more. The path may be right, but the reason for walking this path may be wrong.

Doing good to be happy in life is different from doing good to do well at work. If you choose self-care and it is not for pleasure (for example, you have a massage not to enjoy being present in the experience but to avoid back pain), or you do it so you can work better the next day, then there may be something wrong with your motives. If everything is for work, regret comes, especially if your job is a stressful one that favors the development of humanity's cancer: fear. Fear of not having money, fear of not being able to afford your children's education, fear of not having a place to live. You justify it as "I have to work."

And if you have to do something you do not like, it is because you believe you are helping someone who has not asked for your help. And then how do you justify it when you are in front of the wall? I imagine that on my wall, there is a mirror in which I have to look myself in the eye. "So how did you get here?" I have to explain to myself the path by which I arrived here. I do not have to explain it to my son, to my parents, to my friends. I do not have to explain it to my boss or to my coworkers who wanted to throw me under a bus. In the end, it is me with myself, with no mediators. I need to understand my death because it is mine. The wall of my death is not my son's, my husband's, my father's, my mother's, or my boss's. The path is mine. The matter of work is similar.

Thinking about this may change your life before you become sick, before you really face death. It does not take much time to change your life. The matter of work also appears in matters related to money. Everything you earn for your work also has the same energy you deposit into your work. A few years ago, a nurse friend was promoted to a management position in a large hospital. The only thing I managed to say to her was "Pay attention to what you are going to do with this life that is coming." I could not congratulate her. Knowing how good and pure in heart she was, the life that awaited her would be more full of sorrows and problems than a better-filled bank account. It would be very likely that the extra percentage she would be paid at work would be dedicated to spending on therapy, medicines, and—considering it more seriously—the chemotherapy she needed 2 years later, followed by her funeral.

The energy that comes from work that brings no meaning to your life is bad energy as well. With that money, you will buy food that will spoil faster, you will have a car that will break down all the time, and you will join a gym you will not attend. You will buy clothes you will not wear, and you will pay for courses you will not remember. When you begin to look at your life and everything you can buy is not working well, it may be that the money that is being used does not come from a very good source. I think that you also have to spend money to be able to have the sensation of being alive. If you make a fortune, buy a car, and arrive home looking like a zombie, there is something wrong.

Another regret goes like this: "I should have spent more time with my friends." Since Facebook was born, we feel as though we are with our friends. I am one of those people who have the sensation of being close to friends when I am in front of my Facebook feed. I make good use of this tool and thoroughly enjoy any time I can share with these friends who are so dear to me but so far away. There are people I love dearly, but the life I lead at the moment does not allow me to have a more constant physical presence. I follow their pictures of their children growing, the important moments, the shared tastes, the music and poetry, and somehow I feel part of this parallel universe. At some level, I am actually meeting with these people. But this thing of being with friends, I think, is vital. I feel that with friends, we have a more honest and transparent relationship that is not always possible to live with our families. It is with friends that we have a chance to say, "I didn't like what you did," and we will be fine because they will handle hearing this. When we are with friends, we want to experience this true thing of making our choices and having our feelings respected. People from our families often are not the nicest people in the world, nor ones around whom you want to live.

We can count on our fingers the people who like spending Christmas with their family. Many people spend it with family because they have to, but they do not actually enjoy it. Anyway, being with friends is missed more sorely when we have more free time. Unfortunately, it is when we get sick that we have the most free time. That is why this matter of being with your friends hits you so hard. Then you regret it and think you had free time all your life, but in fact you did not. There are some regrets we may consider a waste of time at the end of life, and that have no use being a topic of suffering. Often you choose a path you did not know would be bad. Now that you know it, you say you are sorry. It is like playing the lottery and saying, "I chose 44, but 45 was drawn. What was I thinking to not choose 45?!" The simple truth is that you did not choose 45 because you chose 44! It is not fair to judge and condemn yourself for past actions with the knowledge you possess now. When the "I should have" or "I could have" drama begins, it is time to grab the mirror and say "Do not trick yourself." You have no right to judge yourself with the knowledge you have now regarding a decision you made 20 or 30 years ago. Back then, you did not have the same information (in terms of the data, the facts, the amounts, and the consequences) to make this more lucid decision that you would make now. Maybe you could say, "Had I known it would go badly, I would have done it differently." But

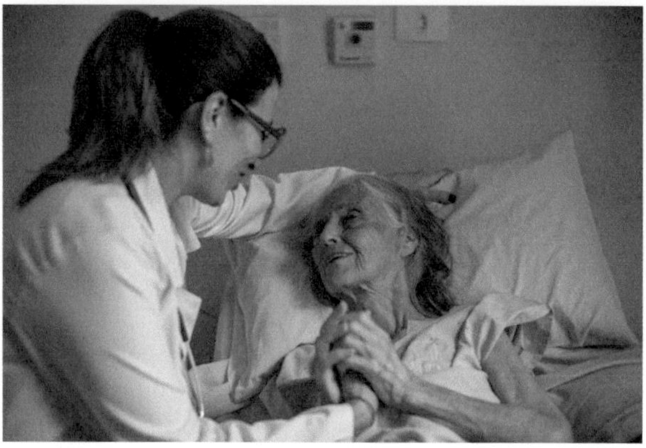

Fig. 9.1 Making oneself happier is related to helping those who are dying and recognizing yourself as an equal

you did not know; there was no way to know how it would be. The proposal of being present in each decision in your life—being present in thoughts, feelings, voice, and attitude—may avoid many of these regrets. At that moment, you make the decision you think best at that moment. Being with friends often makes us experience a state of presence in a joyful way, in an enjoyable way, in a state of consciousness that is full of pleasure and joy, in which we exist entirely in that moment of living it. And often it is friends who offer us this experience.

The last regret—which, in my understanding, sums up all of the others—is "I should have made myself happier." When speaking of the state of happiness, many people think we are talking only about joy and pleasure. But the full state of happiness is often reached after a very hard moment in our lives has been overcome—important and stressful moments we have undergone and out of which we emerged with blood, sweat, and tears, but whole. Covered in scars, but a survivor.

You are better than you were before the hard times started. This brings you a state of full happiness.

Making oneself happier is related to helping someone who is dying and thoroughly looking at that person and recognizing yourself as their equal, because we too are dying. And the most amazing way of helping is being present in that space. When we are helping a person, we are present with them, not within them. And when you can only be in your suffering, you end up using that person to fulfill yourself. What I am saying is cruel, but it is the plain truth. Be careful if you care for someone so you can be someone, using that person to give meaning to your life, be it as a social worker, nurse, physician, child, or spouse. We need compassion to remain in the sacred space of the relationship, of the meeting (Fig. 9.1).

Reference

1. Ware B. The top five regrets of the dying: a life transformed by the dearly departing. London: Hay House; 2011.

Chapter 10
Recommendations for Family Care During Grief

Grief is the response to bereavement, which is the situation in which a loved one has died [1]. The pattern and intensity of grief vary over time as bereaved individuals adapt to the loss. The experience of mourning is influenced by cultural and spiritual rituals, which vary widely, and is unique to each person and each loss. Acute grief can be intense and disturbing, but it ends up being integrated. Progress from acute to integrated grief is often irregular and difficult to discern while it is happening.

Mourning (a process that begins on the day of the loss of a loved one) is one of the most stressful experiences in life. In addition to the loss itself, grief often requires us to redefine goals and plans to restore a meaningful and satisfying life; sometimes there are new responsibilities and roles. Close attachments can possibly be internalized in specific neural networks, and the effects of grief can be measured by changes in these networks [2]. In addition, grieving stress can precipitate or worsen general medical or psychiatric disorders.

Each person who dies leaves behind a variable number of bereaved relatives and friends. People generally have a series of close relationships throughout their lives, which can be depicted with a diagram of concentric circles labeled "acquainted", "closer," and "closest" [3].

There is no standard definition of mourning that identifies who should be considered bereaved. However, close relatives and friends are most affected by a person's death. There are usually between one and five people in the closest group, who are most likely to be profoundly affected by the person's death and are most vulnerable to problems when adapting to the loss (Fig. 10.1).

Grief differs from other adverse events in life, as a period of intense emotional pain and interruption of activities of daily living is expected and socially sanctioned. Although social expectations and ritualization vary widely across cultures, there is generally an expectation that a person will adapt to the loss with adequate support from family and friends [4].

Type of loss Mourning reactions can vary depending on the circumstances of death. In the universe of palliative care, two conditions can prevail:

A. C. L. Q. Arantes, *Clinical Assessment of Human Suffering*,
https://doi.org/10.1007/978-3-030-57535-9_10

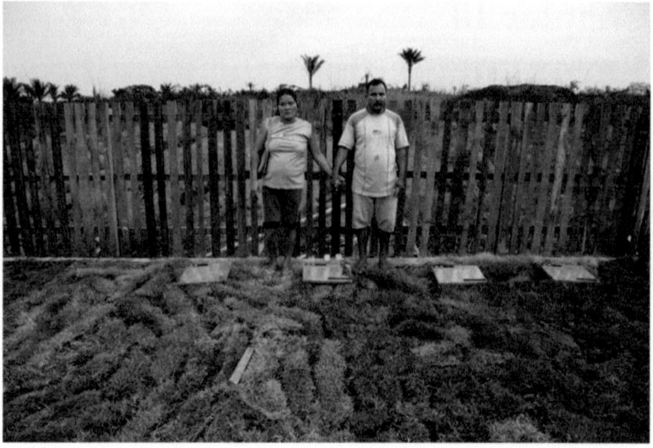

Fig. 10.1 Close relatives and friends are most affected by a person's death

1. *Chronic illness:* When patients die of chronic illness, mourners may have time to anticipate and prepare for the death and begin the process of adaptation. The acute mourning that occurs in response to the loss can be further mitigated in severity or duration. However, chronicity sometimes has the opposite effect; because the disease is long lasting and the patient is still alive, family members may not anticipate the death. In addition, the family's caregiver roles may have predominated and can require an additional level of adaptation after death. Either way, grief often evokes an intense response, even among those whose loss of the loved one is predictable, and psychiatric morbidity can occur.
2. *Terminal illness:* Grief can be preceded by a stressful period of caring for a loved one who is terminally ill; the sensitivity and effectiveness with which terminal illness is treated clinically can affect the caregiver's course of mourning [6–9]. The caregiver's ability to deal with the illness and death of a loved one, as well as the experience of the dying patient, are enhanced by mitigating the patient's suffering; good communication between the medical team and caregivers, and between the caregivers and the dying patient; and preparation for the patient's death.

Use of a hospice can be beneficial, and there is evidence of its impact on the grieving process: use of palliative care by elderly patients may be associated with a decrease in bereavement-related mortality among surviving spouses [10].

Unfortunately, doctors working in palliative care who manage terminal illnesses may not know how to best meet the psychological needs of dying patients and their families. Many clinicians are inexperienced in discussing the prognosis and may experience discomfort with the family's emotional responses [11]. Doctors may overestimate a patient's or family member's understanding of the prognosis and may be unaware of their preferences with regard to receiving this information. Individuals with a low level of preparedness for the death of their spouse have increased risks of anxiety, emotional numbness, and sleep disorders, which can persist for years [12].

The "pyramid" scenario happens when doctors are insensitive or avoid patients who are dying, and caregivers may be at risk of complicated grief and other mental health problems [13].

Mortality Mourning is associated with an increased risk of mortality, after adjustment for chronic medical conditions, access to resources, age, sex, and smoking [14]. Losing a spouse, child, or sibling is associated with an increased risk of death [15].

Complicated grief Grief can lead to complicated grief, which is distinguished from typical acute grief. While acute grief is a natural reaction to the loss of a loved one, complicated grief is a disabling condition in which maladaptive thoughts, feelings, and behaviors interrupt the natural adaptive process and the acute symptoms of grief are intensified and prolonged [16]. The epidemiology, clinical features, assessment, diagnosis, and treatment of complicated grief are discussed elsewhere.

The symptoms of acute grief are typically related to separation from the deceased or to stress and trauma [1, 17].

- Symptoms of separation anguish:
  - Longing for and seeking proximity to the deceased
  - Loneliness
  - Crying, sadness, and other painful emotions (for example, anger, guilt, and anxiety) that occur after being confronted with reminders of the loss
  - Somatic symptoms, including distressing physical sensations and interrupted sleep or appetite
  - Persistent thoughts and memories of the lost person, sometimes including hallucinations
  - Being attracted to things associated with the deceased
  - Social withdrawal and disinterest in other people and activities not associated with the deceased
  - Confusion about identity and feeling lost or uncertain without the deceased
- Trauma/stress reaction symptoms:
  - Disbelief and shock
  - Numbness
  - Impaired attention, concentration, or memory

Some final words In conversation, I can show the person in mourning how the person who died left life full of meaning; after all, the learning and their common story never die. The mourner should never be deprived of their memories and feelings. Love does not die with the physical body. Love always endures. If you have lost or are losing someone you love very much, do this exercise: itemize what you learned from that person and then remember days when you laughed with them. When these memories make you laugh out loud, meditate on that. The tears you shed in that process will greatly alleviate your pain. Tears are made of salt water, like the sea. Crying from that emotion is like bathing in the sea from the inside out.

Everything can die, except for love. Only love deserves immortality within you [18].

References

1. Zisook S, Simon NM, Reynolds CF 3rd, Pies R, Lebowitz B, Young IT, Madowitz J, Shear MK. Bereavement, complicated grief, and DSM, part 2: complicated grief. J Clin Psychiatry. 2010;71(8):1097–8. https://doi.org/10.4088/JCP.10ac06391blu.
2. Stroebe M, Schut H, Stroebe W. Health outcomes of bereavement. Lancet. 2007;370(9603):1960–73. https://doi.org/10.1016/S0140-6736(07)61816-9.
3. Gündel H, O'Connor MF, Littrell L, Fort C, Lane RD. Functional neuroanatomy of grief: an FMRI study. Am J Psychiatry. 2003;160(11):1946–53. https://doi.org/10.1176/appi.ajp.160.11.1946.
4. Antonucci TC, Akiyama H, Takahashi K. Attachment and close relationships across the life span. Attach Hum Dev. 2004;6(4):353–70. https://doi.org/10.1080/1461673042000303136.
5. Zisook S, Shear K. Grief and bereavement: what psychiatrists need to know. World Psychiatry. 2009;8(2):67–74. https://doi.org/10.1002/j.2051-5545.2009.tb00217.x.
6. Schulz R, Boerner K, Shear K, Zhang S, Gitlin LN. Predictors of complicated grief among dementia caregivers: a prospective study of bereavement. Am J Geriatr Psychiatry. 2006;14(8):650–8. https://doi.org/10.1097/01.JGP.0000203178.44894.db.
7. Wright AA, Keating NL, Balboni TA, Matulonis UA, Block SD, Prigerson HG. Place of death: correlations with quality of life of patients with cancer and predictors of bereaved caregivers' mental health. J Clin Oncol. 2010;28(29):4457–64. https://doi.org/10.1200/JCO.2009.26.3863.
8. Tu MS, Chiou CP. Perceptual consistency of pain and quality of life between hospice cancer patients and family caregivers: a pilot study. Int J Clin Pract. 2007;61(10):1686–91. https://doi.org/10.1111/j.1742-1241.2007.01347.x.
9. Chen ML, Chu L, Chen HC. Impact of cancer patients' quality of life on that of spouse caregivers. Support Care Cancer. 2004;12(7):469–75. https://doi.org/10.1007/s00520-004-0636-z.
10. Chiu YW, Huang CT, Yin SM, Huang YC, Chien CH, Chuang HY. Determinants of complicated grief in caregivers who cared for terminal cancer patients. Support Care Cancer. 2010;18(10):1321–7. https://doi.org/10.1007/s00520-009-0756-6.
11. Bradley EH, Prigerson H, Carlson MD, Cherlin E, Johnson-Hurzeler R, Kasl SV. Depression among surviving caregivers: does length of hospice enrollment matter? Am J Psychiatry. 2004;161(12):2257–62. https://doi.org/10.1176/appi.ajp.161.12.2257.
12. Bonanno GA, Papa A, Lalande K, et al. Grief processing and deliberate grief prevention: a prospective comparison of spouses and parents.
13. Kutner JS, Kilbourn KM. Bereavement: addressing challenges faced by advanced cancer patients, their caregivers, and their physicians. Prim Care. 2009;36(4):825–44. https://doi.org/10.1016/j.pop.2009.07.004.
14. Field MJ, Cassel CK, Institute of Medicine Committee on Care at the End of Life. Approaching death: improving care at the end of life. Washington, DC: National Academies Press; 1997.
15. Shah SM, Carey IM, Harris T, DeWilde S, Victor CR, Cook DG. Do good health and material conditions protect the elderly from the increased risk of death after grief? Am J Epidemiol. 2012; 176 (8): 689–698. doi: 10.1093/aje/kws162.
16. Nagraj S, Barclay S. Bereavement care in primary care: a systematic literature review and narrative synthesis. Br J Gen Pract. 2011;61(582):e42–8. https://doi.org/10.3399/bjgp11X549009.
17. Lobb EA, Kristjanson LJ, Aoun SM, Monterosso L, Halkett GK, Davies A. Predictors of complicated grief: a systematic review of empirical studies. Death Stud. 2010;34(8):673–98. https://doi.org/10.1080/07481187.2010.496686.
18. Arantes ACQ. A vida depois da morte: o tempo do luto [Life after death: the time of mourning]. In: Arantes ACQ. A morte é um dia que vale a pena viver [Death is a day worth living]. 2nd edn. Sextante: Sao Paulo; 2019: 175–82.

Chapter 11
The Health Professional Faced with Their Patient's Death: Considerations in Interprofessional Work—The Dimensions of Self-Care

To be considered a caregiver, one must be a health professional who also cares for patients (whether they are hospitalized or not) or a family member, friend, or companion who cares for someone who is in need of any type of care. At this point, it does not matter what type of caregiver you are and whether you are professional or not; what matters is that you know that in order to give care, you need to know who you are very well and why you have chosen to care for someone. Caring is the act of taking care of another person and of yourself. The more whole and present I am in myself, the more ready I am to care for someone.

The health professional is generally overloaded with work, sometimes having to juggle more than two jobs in order to make ends meet. This is a great responsibility, as caring for someone comprises knowing what to do for the health and well-being of that person in need of care. Often it is necessary to live with pain and suffering and, in some cases, with the finitude of life. Often work conditions are not ideal; sometimes the place has inadequate facilities and lacks the ideal number of staff members, materials, and drugs, so the bare minimum will get done. Even if the conditions are not ideal for work, they are ideal for *presence*.

Presence in oneself is a state of deep attention to who you are, the way you feel at that moment, what is happening around you, and how you can actually make a difference in the care of those in need. If you know yourself, you know your own limits, but if you do not know yourself, you might give beyond what you should. When the caregiver gives more than they can, they end up harming their own health, which has biological, emotional, spiritual, social, and family dimensions (Fig. 11.1).

The biological dimension concerns your physical health—having good health and energy for your daily activities. Do you feel active and productive every day? Have you felt any kind of pain or discomfort during the day? When you wake up in the morning, do you feel your sleep was restful or do you feel tired? Are you getting regular exercise? Is your food actually nutritious? Are you going to the doctor regularly? Are your tests up to date? Physical health is very important so that we always have autonomy and vigor to be able to complete all of our daily tasks. Having an

A. C. L. Q. Arantes, *Clinical Assessment of Human Suffering*,
https://doi.org/10.1007/978-3-030-57535-9_11

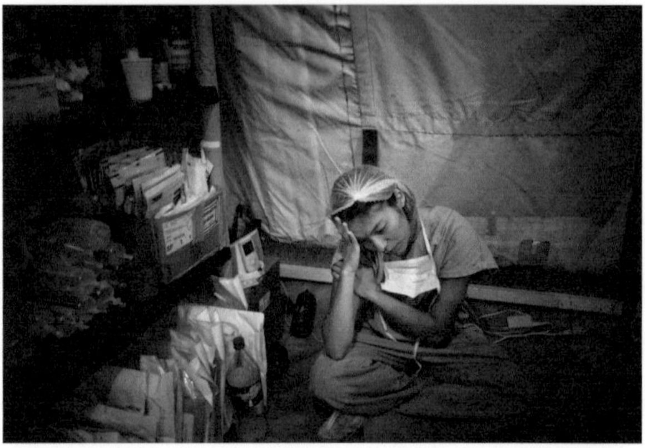

Fig. 11.1 When the caregiver gives more than they can, they end up harming their own health

exercise routine, sleeping well, eating well, observing your body and perceiving what it feels like—whether it is tired or vigorous—these are attitudes we must have as an action goal to reach physical and biological balance.

The emotional dimension concerns how you handle your emotions. Often we cannot control our emotions and end up reacting emotionally. When that occurs, we can have destructive or constructive reactions; how have yours been? Every time you take an attitude on the basis of an emotion, watch and reflect on what you are about to do, and whether it is useful for yourself or for another. Is it useful for the world? What if what you are about to say is true? Is it kind? Is it necessary? The first step in achieving emotional control is to acknowledge what is happening, after recognizing the situation of the emotions you are feeling. Seek to embrace the sensations with no judgment of right or wrong; just observe and embrace them. Investigate this experience and the best way to act in this moment. Often we react automatically to events, but in many instances this reaction is not the most balanced or the one that will produce the best results. Always remember that we must not suppress emotions but simply observe them, take a break, and then take an attitude, with more common sense and peace of mind.

The spiritual dimension concerns your spirituality. What does spirituality mean to you? Spirituality is everything that makes us feel connected, that makes us feel we are part of a larger whole. You can seek this connection through religion but not necessarily only through religion. It may be through nature, looking at a flower, watching a bird, listening to the sound of the sea, walking into a waterfall, strolling through the woods or on a beach—whatever you enjoy the most in contact with nature. Even if you cannot have this contact, know that just looking at a picture of nature or imagining a natural landscape boosts our immune system. We can also access spirituality through the arts—for example, by listening to a song, dancing, singing, writing, writing poetry, painting a picture, playing an instrument, watching an orchestra play, or anything else that makes you feel that you are spiritually nurtured.

The social dimension concerns the way you are inserted into the community where you live and how you socialize with the people in this community. How do you interact with the people who live with you in this community? Do you take part in actions that help make this community better? Do you feel you can make a difference in your community through your actions? Can you create bonds with the people in places you usually visit? Do you contact your friends regularly to chat or meet? It is also very important to have a social activity that gives you pleasure and joy. Interacting with other people can be welcoming and a lot of fun.

The family dimension concerns the way you interact with your family, how important family bonds are to you, how much of your time you spare to be with this family, and the quality of that time. This family can be your blood relations or your chosen family. Is there affection in these relationships? How do you express your affection? Have you had the time to travel or go out with your family? Family relationships are not always easy and often come loaded with emotional burdens, but there is always time to re-evaluate the relationships and how much we can improve them. Sometimes a simple tight hug, a phone call during the day, or a goodnight kiss can rescue once-forgotten affection.

It is very important that these dimensions are in balance, a dynamic balance where we must observe which of them is the most debilitated and which is the most balanced. At each moment in life, we have different needs, but observation and reflection on how we are dealing with each of them is part of the process of autonomy and consciousness we want to develop. Every human being should question all of these aspects, but the health professional or caregiver needs to be well to be able to practice their profession. Knowing who you are, which aspects of your life can be better, and how you feel in all of these dimensions are questions that should be asked daily. Of course, we expect institutions to take care of their employees, but this is not always feasible. What can we do then? As Gandhi said, "Be the change you want to see in the world." In self-observation and self-care, our relationship with ourselves and the way we react to the external world keeps changing; thus, everything around us also changes. Look at yourself and ask, "How much do I keep in me of the pleasure and the love I felt when I first started doing what I chose to do? What makes me feel happy for being alive? What is my purpose in life?" We need some time to reflect on our choices, on the paths we are choosing to walk. We need to turn off cruise control and choose who we actually want to be! We are responsible for the path we walk and predominantly for how we walk that path.

The greatest villains in all of this are stress and the idea that we have to be happy all the time. How do we not get sick while caring for sick people and witnessing so much suffering? Well-being has to do with being resilient, because we are not going to find a perfect world. According to its dictionary definitions, resilience is the ability some bodies have to return to their original form after being subjected to elastic deformation, or the capacity to return to a natural state after a situation of difficulty or great stress. But in order to return to our state of well-being, we need to know what state that is. If we live in stress, running against the clock, reacting to each and every external event, how can we go back to our original state if we don't even know who we really are? The less stress we have, the fewer gifts we have. Chronic stress dehumanizes us and creates a protective shell.

> Forget about enlightenment.
> Sit down wherever you are
> And listen to the wind singing in your veins.
> Feel the love, the longing, the fear in your bones.
> Open your heart to who you are, right now,
> Not who you would like to be,
> Not the saint you are striving to become,
> But the being right here before you, inside you, around you.
> All of you is holy.
> You are already more and less
> Than whatever you can know.
> Breathe out,
> Touch in,
> Let go.
>
> (John Welwood)

Chapter 12
Caring for Caregivers

The world: planet Earth. We live here, we work here, we are health professionals, and we are human. The latest statistics regarding human mortality on our planet show that of the 56.9 million deaths that occurred worldwide in 2016, more than half (54%) were related to ten diseases (Table 12.1), which, in their natural course, cause suffering in all dimensions—physical, emotional, family, social, and spiritual—despite all available treatments. These diseases have remained the principal causes of global death for the last 15 years, and it is worth mentioning that these statistics refer to officially diagnosed causes of death; that is, these people were diagnosed with diseases that threaten the continuity of life, and they would therefore have been candidates to receive palliative care [1].

Like me, millions of health professionals need to take care of people—of human beings—in an unbearable degree of suffering throughout this year. Certainly, the vast majority of people die under very poor care received from health professionals who have never been adequately trained to support and assist people who die. For each of these human beings who die, there are many stories and moments, much sadness, much unresolved pain, and good and bad words, spoken and unspoken, that wander through the memories of those who remain. For the relatives and loved ones

Table 12.1 The top ten causes of death in the world in 2016 [1]

Cause
1. Ischemic heart disease
2. Cerebrovascular accident
3. Chronic obstructive pulmonary disease
4. Infections of the lower respiratory tract
5. Alzheimer's disease and other mental illnesses
6. Lung, trachea, and bronchial cancer
7. Diabetes mellitus
8. Traffic accidents
9. Diarrheal diseases
10. Tuberculosis

A. C. L. Q. Arantes, *Clinical Assessment of Human Suffering*,
https://doi.org/10.1007/978-3-030-57535-9_12

of these people who die, we expect the pain of mourning, which is recognized by society as legitimate. Fathers, mothers, children, siblings, spouses, friends—everyone can cry for their dead. But there are many tears lost in the rain. The suffering of the health professionals who take care of these people is not recognized, or legitimized, or even allowed in our culture of health care (or, rather, illness).

Countless undergraduate health courses in the world provide entry into a labor market in a world of pain, aging, death, suffering, and losses—both tangible and intangible—that surround and occupy the entire space of people's lives when they lose their health. We start our training with dreams of curing *diseases*, but what we find in reality is that we are not prepared to care for *people* who are sick. We receive preparation for dealing with the disease, but we do not realize that the biggest difficulty is dealing with those who are sick. Worse, we do not realize that because we are as human as our patients, suffering hits our small personal world in such an overwhelming way that we are often swallowed up by it. The usual coping strategy recommended by those who are more experienced is that we should not get involved. I understand that to be considered more experienced, professionals need to be recognized as strong, and being strong in the ignorant translation of our culture is the same as being tough, insensitive, and alienated from the suffering of those around you. But, as life is generous and patient, time will teach these "strong" professionals that the pain is unbearable even for them.

One who throws stones will be the glass house at some point in their life. I do not say this with the intention of reprisal or punishment, as our human condition will certainly lead us to experience gradual or sudden losses of functions, of goods, of social positions, of autonomy, and also of people we love. Believe me, those who are cruel also love, and for love, they too suffer. And through their pain, they will be able to understand what it means to suffer without care.

The health professional who is sensitive to their surroundings of suffering appears to be a person at severe risk of professional burnout. In my years of taking care of critically ill patients, observing the evolution of each one at the end of life, I have realized that everything is like a great gift. The biggest lesson for all of us is that life is nothing but a great gift. It is not yesterday, nor tomorrow. It is not a burden nor a prize. It is present; it is now. The chance to be with those who are departing from this life is given to each of us—mainly because we will all depart. The awareness of finitude should always be present because it is this wisdom that allows us to perceive life as unique and so special. Death is a great specialist in teaching us about priorities, as it allows us the awareness that can ensure that life is lived to its fullest.

Death is denied and avoided, but it really should not be seen as a bad witch or a skull armed with a scythe and looking like Friday the 13th. Saramago [2] has already shown us how difficult life would be if death were saddened by its fame. Perhaps death is like a fairy who can transform our last days into better days, as long as we wish for it. Transforming last moments into eternal moments—perhaps the best moments—is death's great purpose, because death can exist only to give meaning to life.

We all have personal issues that we try to postpone until a time far from the present moment. We even have pains that we believe will never be cured. By reserving for our final moments a series of decisions and actions that we have postponed for a lifetime, we have the impression that we have moved away from these wounds. But as we approach our end, these pains beg for healing and relief. We can then take care of and answer this call in a much more serene way, as this is one of the gifts that death brings us: serenity. But as we are not sure that we will have the chance to know that we are living our last moments, we take a risk. We risk the possibility of fullness in our day, as we always leave aside some fulfillment, some difficult conversation, a request for forgiveness, a declaration of love.

The awareness of our ending must guarantee for us that in every moment of our lives, we are doing our best. Surrender at each moment that is experienced can reverse much of what we call regret. In general, we are driven by a force toward the future; at other times, we are justified only by what has happened to us in the past. We can be bound with strong chains or, conversely, we can be holding those chains, believing that they are what bind us. Releasing the chains that hold you back can be very challenging and fearful, but it can also mean the freedom to live untethered in the present moment, available for what it has to offer.

This life is unique; this experience now is unique. It will not be repeated.

Even if you read this sentence a thousand times, the first time will be different from the thousandth. Time does not repeat itself. Stories seem to repeat themselves, but in fact they are unique in each moment when they take place. For it does not matter what your beliefs are or whether you are an atheist, but it is certain that in this life, here and now, we pass only once. There may be others, or not, but here and now, we pass only once. There may be life after death, life after life, but life now is unique and singular. It would be very interesting if we could make the best of every moment of this opportunity.

So it seems to me that a care team is insensitive to the final moments of a human being. It offers an endless bondage of suffering, simply postponing what is already known to be inevitable. And the suffering offered to patients who are in the final stages of life and undergoing all sorts of futile procedures may be short lived, but it will always bring the impression of having lasted 100 years. Pleasure is always short lived, but unbearable pain that lasts for any time will always seem eternal.

Unfortunately, in college we did not learn that life is much more than biological survival.

We are alongside our patient; we do not walk past them. We do not feel their pain, but we know how to relieve it. We do not live the loss that they live, but we should focus on helping them transcend the loss and rediscover strength and the infinite capacity to smile and feel good, despite everything (Fig. 12.1).

Humans beings are complex beings, gifted with multiple impressions regarding the world and themselves, learned and incorporated into their way of living and thinking throughout their lives. At birth, we are essentially a biological being, but as we grow older, our biographical dimension is enriched. And our suffering dimension goes way beyond suffering from physical illness. Cats are born cats, and each one believes it is the only one to exist, for it does not know the stories of other cats. If it gets sick, it has no sense of suffering from finitude, because it is oblivious to the natural history of life.

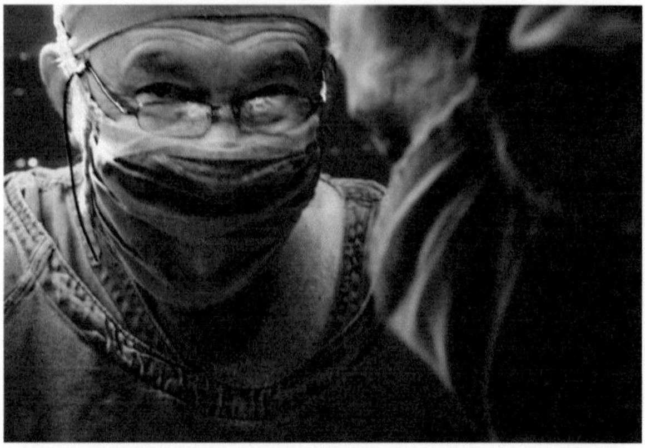

Fig. 12.1 The physician's life is as important and valuable as all of the lives they are dedicated to caring for

As human beings grow, we learn stories of the lives of other human beings. Some diseases already have a well-recorded history in the collective unconscious as facades of the end of life. Just knowing about a diagnosis—of cancer, for example—makes us think about the threat to our integrity. Other diseases still in disguise, such as diabetes and heart failure, carry in themselves great gravity but cover up their importance and deprive their carriers of knowing how much they can threaten them.

Often, in the case of health professionals, the absence of a physical disease does not mean the absence of suffering. And in the vast majority of cases, health professionals' malaise begins in their professional dimension, then the emotional one, hurting a family member, taking away their spiritual sense, until, finally, they succumb to physical illness.

The comprehensive task for physicians is to analyze and act on diseases in accordance with their patients' preferences in order to ensure better-integrated conversations in medical consultations and greater attention to psychosocial issues and the problems involved. The final challenge is not cognitive but behavioral: maintaining close contact with the clinician's own humanity, no matter how stressful their day is, and connecting with the patient. The increasing prevalence of burnout among doctors can make it more difficult to be emotionally present in the moment with a patient [1].

This behavioral task of establishing a good connection with each patient must be realistically considered within the context of consultations of a limited duration in doctors' offices and hospitals. Research shows that expressly attending to problems laden with emotions can, in fact, improve efficiency, patient satisfaction, and professional satisfaction [3]. Approaches that have been proven to save time include allowing patients to offer and complete their opening statements, negotiating an agreed and prioritized agenda for the meeting, responding to patients' reactions and concerns with empathy, and providing patient guidance regarding the events occurring during the meeting [4].

The drama of burnout within the universe of health professionals is more frequent than we would like. Burnout syndrome is characterized by loss of enthusiasm for work (emotional exhaustion), treating people as if they were objects (depersonalization), and feeling that work is no longer significant (poor personal achievement) [6]. Numerous global studies involving almost all medical and surgical specialties indicate that approximately one in three doctors experiences burnout at some time [5].

The prevalence of burnout among physicians is a cause for concern. Exhaustion seems to alter both the doctor–patient relationship and the quality of care provided by doctors. The doctor's wear and tear also seem to influence patient adherence to recommended therapy, the degree of trust the patient has in their doctor, and patient satisfaction with medical care [6]. In addition to these professional repercussions, burnout can have profound personal consequences for doctors, including substance abuse, a desire to abandon medical practice, and suicide [5, 7].

The factors that contribute to the wear and tear of the doctor are complex. Most studies consider loss of autonomy, a reduction in control over the practice environment, and inefficient use of time, due to administrative requirements, to be central factors [5]. Other research has implicated the workload, choice of specialty, establishment of practices, sleep deprivation, lack of balance between professional and personal life, medical errors, the risk of malpractice proceedings, the characteristics of treated patients, and the methods used by doctors to deal with patients' deaths and illnesses as contributing factors [5]. These variables interact in unique ways, depending on the personal responsibilities of each doctor, their personality, their coping strategies, and other factors, which are probably responsible for the variations in stress among doctors in similar professional circumstances [8].

Other studies have suggested that promoting self-awareness can help doctors to identify what they value and to connect with what is most significant in their work [9]. A variety of methods can be used to help promote awareness and reflection. For example, doctors may be asked to reflect or write a short narrative about a specific personal experience in their practice (for example, being with a patient at the end of their life, making a medical error, or remembering a particularly significant encounter), with a focus on how they reacted and worked with the situation [10, 11]. Participants can share their experience (and listen to other people's experiences) with a small group of colleagues, who listen with the intention of understanding the speaker's experience rather than interpreting or judging it [10]. The whole process of self-care should convey to the health professional that their life is as important and valuable as all of the lives they are dedicated to caring for. Therefore, it should receive the same attention to—and care for—its own human dimensions: physical, emotional, family, social, and spiritual. With this care, we can then dedicate ourselves in a more conscious way and become more capable of achieving the results that we long for in our work.

References

1. Shanafelt TD. Enhancing meaning in work: a prescription for preventing physician burnout and promoting patient-centered care. JAMA. 2009;302(12):1338–40. https://doi.org/10.1001/jama.2009.1385.
2. Saramago J. As intermitências da morte [Death at intervals]. Lisbon: Círculo de Leitores; 2006.
3. Panagioti M, Panagopoulou E, Bower P, Lewith G, Kontopantelis E, Chew-Graham C, Dawson S, van Marwijk H, Geraghty K, Esmail A. Controlled interventions to reduce burnout in physicians: a systematic review and meta-analysis. JAMA Intern Med. 2017;177(2):195–205. https://doi.org/10.1001/jamainternmed.2016.7674.
4. Roter DL, Stewart M, Putnam SM, Lipkin M Jr, Stiles W, Inui TS. Communication patterns of primary care physicians. JAMA. 1997;277(4):350–6. https://doi.org/10.1001/jama.1997.03540280088045.
5. Shanafelt TD, Sloan JA, Habermann TM. The well-being of physicians. Am J Med. 2003;114(6):513–9. https://doi.org/10.1016/s0002-9343(03)00117-7.
6. DiMatteo MR, Sherbourne CD, Hays RD, Ordway L, Kravitz RL, McGlynn EA, Kaplan S, Rogers WH. Physicians' characteristics influence patients' adherence to medical treatment: results from the Medical Outcomes Study. Health Psychol. 1993;12(2):93–102. https://doi.org/10.1037/0278-6133.12.2.93.
7. Dyrbye LN, Thomas MR, Massie FS, Power DV, Eacker A, Harper W, Durning S, Moutier C, Szydlo DW, Novotny PJ, Sloan JA, Shanafelt TD. Burnout and suicidal ideation among US medical students. Ann Intern Med. 2008;149(5):334–41. https://doi.org/10.7326/0003-4819-149-5-200809020-00008.
8. Linzer M, Visser MR, Oort FJ, Smets EM, McMurray JE, de Haes HC. Society of General Internal Medicine (SGIM) Career Satisfaction Study Group (CSSG). Predicting and preventing physician burnout: results from the United States and the Netherlands. Am J Med. 2001;111(2):170–5. https://doi.org/10.1016/s0002-9343(01)00814-2.
9. Epstein RM. Mindful practice. JAMA. 1999;282(9):833–9. https://doi.org/10.1001/jama.282.9.833.
10. Rabow MW, McPhee SJ. Doctoring to heal: fostering well-being among physicians through personal reflection. West J Med. 2001;174(1):66–9. https://doi.org/10.1136/ewjm.174.1.66.
11. McCue JD, Sachs CL. A stress management workshop improves residents' coping skills. Arch Intern Med. 1991;151(11):2273–7. https://doi.org/10.1001/archinte.1991.00400110117023.

Index

A. C. L. Q. Arantes, *Clinical Assessment of Human Suffering*,
https://doi.org/10.1007/978-3-030-57535-9

MIX
Papier aus verantwortungsvollen Quellen
Paper from responsible sources
FSC® C105338

If you have any concerns about our products,
you can contact us on
ProductSafety@springernature.com

In case Publisher is established outside the EU,
the EU authorized representative is:
Springer Nature Customer Service Center GmbH
Europaplatz 3, 69115 Heidelberg, Germany

Printed by Libri Plureos GmbH
in Hamburg, Germany